T0386142

MIND, MOOD, AND MEMORY

MIND, MOOD, AND MEMORY

The Neurobehavioral Consequences of Multiple Sclerosis

ANTHONY FEINSTEIN

Foreword by Alan Thompson, MD

JOHNS HOPKINS UNIVERSITY PRESS | *Baltimore*

Johns Hopkins University Press
2715 North Charles Street
Baltimore, Maryland 21218-4363
www.press.jhu.edu

Library of Congress Cataloging-in-Publication Data

Names: Feinstein, A. (Anthony), 1956– author.
Title: Mind, mood, and memory : the neurobehavioral consequences
    of multiple sclerosis / Anthony Feinstein ; foreword by Alan Thompson, MD.
Description: Baltimore : Johns Hopkins University Press, 2022. |
    Includes bibliographical references and index.
Identifiers: LCCN 2021018588 | ISBN 9781421443232 (hardcover) |
    ISBN 9781421443249 (ebook)
Subjects: LCSH: Multiple sclerosis—Psychological aspects. |
    Multiple sclerosis—Complications. | Clinical neuropsychology.
Classification: LCC RC377 .F45 2022 | DDC 616.8/34—dc23
LC record available at https://lccn.loc.gov/2021018588

A catalog record for this book is available from the British Library.

Special discounts are available for bulk purchases of this book. For more
information, please contact Special Sales at specialsales@jh.edu.

To Maria Ron

"Example is not the main thing in influencing others. It is the only thing."

—Albert Schweitzer

CONTENTS

Compared to the past, it is more common today to recognize and to discuss many of the neurobehavioral effects of multiple sclerosis, including cognitive impairment and mood disorders. However, this increased awareness doesn't necessarily mean that these disorders are assessed in routine neurological practice or, indeed, effectively managed.

In his book, *Mind, Mood, and Memory: The Neurobehavioral Consequences of Multiple Sclerosis*, Anthony Feinstein introduces us to the wide-ranging components of the complex picture of cognitive impairment and mood disorders associated with MS. He graphically, and sometimes uncomfortably, describes how these disorders affect individuals, while providing an understanding of mechanistic underpinnings and insights into how best to assess the behavioral changes and develop solutions for them.

The book moves from specific deficits, such as those involving processing speed, learning, and memory, to broader, more complex issues, such as irritability, sadness, and the unraveling of personality, which I found particularly illuminating. The book builds a coherent picture of the increasingly devastating impact these deficits have on the person affected by MS and even more so on those who love, and live with, them.

The content and style of this important work are equally matched in providing a comprehensive and accessible narrative that educates and informs. All aspects of mind, mood, and memory are addressed, and this is done in a logical and cumulative way that is both interesting and informative. Feinstein manages to weave in the myriad cognitive tests in a way that makes perfect sense and, therefore, makes them surprisingly easy to remember. The research insights add depth and raise important questions that will stimulate the reader and encourage further exploration.

Each chapter is brought to life by the impactful case histories used to illustrate the real-world consequences of cognitive impairments and mood disorders. Rather than draw on real-life individuals, which is what might be expected, Feinstein has drawn on his vast experience to create characters with particular circumstances. One might think this approach wouldn't work and that the characters might seem "unreal" or wooden. But the very opposite is true; it is often unbearably sad. What makes the crucial difference is the graphic style in which they are presented. You can visualize the individuals and their families, and the consultations are brought to life with vivid descriptions of peoples' appearances, demeanors, and concerns.

That brings me neatly to the style of the writing, which is both accomplished and immediate. Feinstein writes with an easy and relaxed style, sprinkling his narrative with quotes and aphorisms. How extraordinary to begin with Churchill but how apposite—"to know how to command the moment to remain"—to remain in the present and take what is on offer, a point that resonates throughout the book. His description of the impact of MS as "slowing life to a shuffle in an ever-smaller orbit" is accurate and poignant, and it is complemented by the Philip Roth quote that "life is a complicated business, fraught with mystery and some sunshine"—to which Feinstein adds, "welcome to the world of a person with MS." Some of his descriptors are powerful and the images they convey devastating. When talking about the effect of reduced processing speed on one patient who had exhausted her compensatory skills, he quotes her as saying, "the lemon had been squeezed dry." Later, he describes a pair of pristine shoes, a touching marker of disability in a particular individual who was no longer able to walk. There are many such astute observations—pithy and pertinent—throughout the book.

Overall this is a comprehensive, stimulating read that is accessible and instructive. It flows easily and naturally and the only times I had to stop reading was when I became overwhelmed by the cruel and relentless impact of cognitive impairment and mood disorders on people with MS and their families. The book underlines the impact at every turn and by implication emphasizes the need for greater understanding and better management of the multiple deficits that accompany this disease. By the end, there is little of this hidden disability that has not been uncovered.

This book is essential reading for anyone who wants to understand the impact cognitive impairment and emotional dysregulation, in all their forms, have on people with MS and on those who support them. And how appropriate that Feinstein has dedicated his book to Maria Ron, someone from whom we, in the MS world, have learned a great deal and who has done so much to raise the profile of cognitive impairment in MS.

Alan Thompson, MD
Dean, Faculty of Brain Sciences
and Pro-Provost for London
University College London

MIND, MOOD, AND MEMORY

Introduction

THERE ARE MORE than 2.5 million people worldwide with multiple sclerosis. The majority of those with MS will not become severely disabled and two-thirds will remain able to walk. For those who are doing well and have mild disability, a yearly check-in with their neurologist will be all that is required medically. A brief history is taken, a neurological examination is performed, and an MRI is undertaken to determine whether there are imaging signs of disease activity. And then, all being well, the next appointment is booked for the following year.

When you work in a specialist neuropsychiatry clinic within a tertiary care hospital, you see a different side to the disease. To be sure, there is still a group of people with MS who are managing well, whose disease is mild or moderate in severity, and whose appointments need be no more frequent than once or twice a year. But there is another, larger, group who are having a very tough time with a very tough disease. Given that I run a neuropsychiatry service, the people who come to see me are generally battling an array of behavioral difficulties, such as cognitive dysfunction, depression, anxiety, pseudobulbar affect, and apathy, disorders which are not mutually exclusive. Often, these people also have major physical challenges, but not invariably so. Should you take a seat in my waiting room on any given day, there will be times when you may be forgiven in doubting whether the clinic specializes in MS at all. For people will walk in and out, unaided and seemingly in robust health. But appearances can be deceptive. Loss of memory, slowed processing speed, and crippling depression, to mention but three common presentations, are invisible to the naked eye. They are part of a hidden disability that occurs in many people with MS, and these symptoms can bring a person down very hard indeed. My book tells their stories.

Writing about one's patients is challenging, particularly from a mental health perspective, for there are many small intimacies divulged and painful, private feelings laid bare. A psychiatrist asking for permission to expose these confidences places the person with MS in a difficult, conflictual situation—on the one hand wanting to help the therapist who is helping them, on the other wanting to maintain personal confidentiality and privacy. These competing desires are often irreconcilable and, in terms of priorities, the desire to maintain privacy comes first. There is also the risk that in asking for permission to divulge a person's medical, psychiatric, family, and personal histories, the clinician may disrupt the therapeutic alliance that has formed.

Mindful of these pitfalls, I have adopted a different approach to the case histories in this book. I have used poetic license to create the individuals whose emotional, cognitive, and behavioral difficulties I describe. I have run an MS neuropsychiatry clinic for going on 30 years. During that time, thousands of people with MS attending my service have been assessed, treated, and discharged. Their life stories, each unique, also have a common thread, which is the challenge presented by living well with MS. By reworking, modifying, altering, combining, trimming, expanding, and reinventing the gist of these real-life stories, I have created the fictional people who populate these case histories. This has freed me from the constraints that come with disclosure. What often gives psychiatric histories their power to move a person are those personal, intimate details around which a life pivots and a future is decided. Not being able to share them can weaken the narrative and ensure that one falls short in conveying to the reader the enormity of the challenges faced by many people with MS as they navigate the choppy waters of their disease.

If poetic license characterizes the fictional people with MS portrayed in my book, no such liberty has been adopted in my review of the current state of the neuropsychiatry literature. This is not meant to be an exhaustive overview of what is now a large and rapidly expanding field. Rather, the references have been chosen with an eye to the case histories. There is much research still to be done, but there is already a sizable amount of good, sound scientific evidence that can help clinicians gain a better understanding of the neuropsychiatric difficulties that come with MS. It is my hope that, by marrying these two approaches, the unadorned facts of the disease are brought to life by reconstructed narratives which reveal the myriad challenges, successes, failures, heartaches, and joys that come from living with MS.

ONE

The Paradox of Time and Space

ON A VISIT to Italy in the immediate aftermath of World War II, Winston Churchill imparted some simple yet profound wisdom on two junior officers who had been assigned to his security detail. "Out of a life of long and varied experience," he told them, "the most valuable piece of advice I could hand on to you is to know how to command the moment to remain."[1]

Churchill was 70 years of age at the time. It is remarkable that a man whose life had been defined by such prodigious energy, constant action, derring-do, relentless travel, and perpetual movement should distill from it such an insight, in a sense the antithesis of all that had preceded it. To be sure, Churchill's moment of quiet reflection was prompted by a site of rare beauty as he sat looking out over the still waters of Lake Como on a warm late summer's evening.

The reader could be forgiven for asking what relevance this anecdote has for people with multiple sclerosis. What lesson are they to take from the hero of the hour contemplating a vista of sublime serenity after years of terrible conflict? Apart from the more obvious superficial association of prolonged battles as a metaphor for a lengthy, debilitating illness, the pleasure of contemplating Lake Como is a world away from the grim reality of a walker or wheelchair. What they share, however, is asking the individual to remain present and to take what is on offer, surely a more pleasurable challenge in the case of Lake Como. But for the disabled person with MS, the stakes are indisputably much higher, for the desire to flee the moment, to blot out thoughts of what might have been, and to take refuge in denial and the past will ensure a life that never catches up to reality.

People with MS who become physically and cognitively disabled have to confront and prevail over a world that closes in around them, shrinking in space and time. How they overcome this inordinately difficult hurdle will define their lives. Solitude becomes disability's companion, if one lets it. The adjustment to this new, unsolicited reality can prove the greatest challenge of living with MS. Time and again I have seen how a busy life has slowed and contracted, the horizon creeping inexorably closer.

The criteria for diagnosing multiple sclerosis have changed over time. The Schumacher criteria[2] (1965) gave way to the Poser criteria[3] (1983), which in turn were supplanted by the McDonald criteria[4] (2001), which have since undergone multiple revisions.[5-7] What has remained constant across the decades, even as technology has raced ahead, is the core clinical principle that defines the disorder, the bedrock on which all the technological advances rest. I refer to evidence of damage to the central nervous system that is disseminated in space and time. And therein lies a paradox.

Let us start with time. For most people with MS, time brings with it new and worsening symptoms, a bigger lesion load, increasing brain atrophy, and greater disability. Even in the age of disease-modifying drugs, the ticking clock can portend physical and cognitive decline as clinically isolated syndromes give way to relapsing-remitting disease, followed by a secondary progressive course (figure 1.1[8,9]). One in five people with MS will be using a cane within 15 years of diagnosis,[10] 48% of those receiving home care require a wheelchair,[11] and MS will shorten a person's lifespan by around seven years.[12] The paradox for people with MS is that time-dependent disability is associated with time slowing in their personal lives. As disability mounts, activities lessen, work is lost,

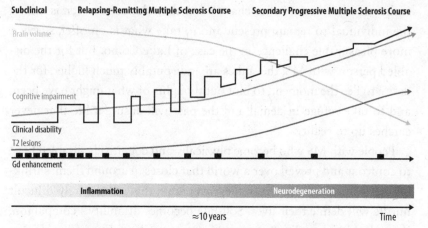

Figure 1.1. Increasing disability with dissemination of damage to the central nervous system over time. Gd = Gadolinium (contrast enhanced). Image courtesy of Biogen; see refs. 8 and 9 in chap. 1.

friendships fall away, leisure pursuits are curtailed, and slowly, relentlessly, life decelerates and, with it, time does as well. A life stripped of activities changes its relationship with time. Days drag by interminably. "Time is created by events," observed Berger and Demirel—the disabled person, marooned by a faltering gait or sieve-like memory knows only too well from personal experience that "time is much kinder at night . . . [for] there's nothing to wait for."[13] The *New Oxford Thesaurus of English* lists a number of synonyms for *dissemination*. Dispersal, diffusion, spreading, passing on, all applicable to central nervous system damage and disease progression but the very antithesis of the external time-tethered reality that disabled people confront in their daily lives. More apt is "stifled in time." Juxtaposed like this, one-half of the paradox is starkly revealed.

The other half of the paradox pertains to space, of lesions disseminated in numerous locations across the central nervous system. This, too, is essential when it comes to diagnosing MS. The use of magnetic resonance imaging (MRI) has been pivotal in demonstrating this characteristic disease phenomenon. But as the brain atrophies and the space occupied by MS lesions increases with time, typically encompassing the optic nerves and periventricular, brain stem, and cerebellar regions, so the space linked to a person's daily activities shrinks (see figure 1.1). When work is no longer possible, there is no office to go to. As walking falters, socializing becomes more of a challenge and the homes of friends and family are closed off. Public spaces are the next to go. Favorite haunts are abandoned because they are no longer accessible. In time, as disability mounts, the cumulative effects of pain, spasticity, and incontinence create an ever-larger barrier to engaging with the world hurrying by. At some point for many people with MS, the simple mechanics of getting around proves so wearing it becomes preferable to stay at home. But even here space is shrinking. Staircases curtail movement, but finances are now limited for work has stopped, so the solution of giving up the current house for a single-level home is not possible. And one cannot simply rearrange the house by shifting a bedroom downstairs when there is no bathroom on the ground floor and no money to install one. So it goes, one space after another blocked off, the world shrinking piecemeal. To be sure, there are outings to the shops, the mall, and the cinema from time to time, but these dwindle too, especially when friendships are lost and parents age. The world closes in. Space, a commodity so prized and sought after, contracts. All the while, lesions continue to multiply throughout the brain and spinal cord, occupying more space—a constant reminder of the paradox inherent to the diagnosis: Dissemination in time and space, slowing life to a shuffle in an ever-smaller orbit.

At every step along the Via Dolorosa to increasing disability, Churchill's advice rings true. Command the moment to remain. As we will read in later chapters, the temptation to lessen the distress of a stymied life by avoiding the moment can be overwhelming. So, too, the temptation to rail against it, the unfairness of it all, the randomness of fate dealing one a bad hand. But, as we shall see, there are ways to move forward and lessen the burden of this unforgiving disease. Planning and strategizing, with the help of a psychotherapist or occupational therapist, open the door to an improved quality of life. Horizons can expand once more and with them the tempo of life quickens. But first, to get the process started, to begin the return journey, comes acceptance, and for that, the person with MS must learn how to command the moment to remain. An extraordinarily difficult task. But not impossible.

TWO

Cognition in General and Processing Speed in Particular

THE NINETEENTH-CENTURY French neurologist Jean-Martin Charcot was the most perceptive of clinicians. Testimony to this can be found in the numerous medical syndromes and clinical signs that now carry his name.* He left his mark in the domain of MS too—the Charcot neurologic triad, referring to nystagmus, intention tremor, and dysarthria, all signs of cerebellar involvement. Perhaps less well-known are his behavioral observations of his MS patients. Almost 150 years ago, he noted that some showed a "marked feebleness of the memory, conceptions are formed slowly and intellectual and emotional faculties are blunted in their totality."[1] History reveals that he was well ahead of his peers here. With a few notable exceptions, little further was published on the subject for over a century. It took one of the great advances in medicine, the arrival of magnetic resonance imaging (MRI), to change all that. The first MRI in a person with MS was performed in 1981 in England, and it provided a window into the brain. Significantly superior to computerized

---

* Such was Charcot's fame at the time, he even had an island in Antarctica named after him, courtesy of his explorer son, who would from time to time attend his father's clinical presentations at the Salpêtrière Hospital in Paris.

axial tomography (CT) in visualizing brain anatomy and the telltale plaques that characterize the disease, MRI galvanized clinical and research interest in multiple sclerosis.

The potential clinical significance of the remarkable images that began appearing on MRI consoles was not lost on behavioral scientists. And for those with a penchant for history, the observations of Charcot were dusted off, quoted anew, and given fresh impetus by a safe imaging technique that provided the wherewithal to understand the mechanisms underpinning a "feeble" memory. What followed was an outpouring of research devoted to the behavioral consequences of a disease that is the commonest cause of neurological disability in young and middle-aged adults.

Ten years on from the first MRI in a person with MS, a seminal neuropsychological paper by Rao et al. revealed that 43% of people with the disease were cognitively impaired.[2] The result was quickly replicated.[3] This figure, derived from extensive neuropsychological testing, was almost nine times the estimate based on a neurological examination.[4] Indeed, subsequent research showed that neurologists without recourse to cognitive testing were no more accurate than chance when it came to determining the presence of cognitive dysfunction.[5] What is equally telling is that 30 years on from Rao and colleagues' landmark paper, the overall estimate of global impairment still holds true. What has changed in the interim, however, is an appreciation of prevalence figures differing according to disease course. Thus, while the rate of impairment in relapsing-remitting MS is estimated at 45%, this may increase to approximately 80% in secondary progressive disease and 90% in primary progressive MS. Even in people with clinically isolated syndromes (CIS), frequently the precursor to MS, impairment is present in a third of individuals.[6] A similar percentage of people with a radiologically isolated syndrome (RIS)—namely, the absence of neurological symptoms but with an MRI suggestive of MS—will be affected.[7] This increase in frequency and severity of cognitive deficits from disease onset to 4 and 10 years thereafter has been clearly defined in two informative longitudinal studies from Maria Pia Amato's group in Florence.[8,9] It is now also evident that isolated cognitive relapses can occur, unrelated to depression, fatigue, and subjective cognitive complaints, in neurologically stable people with relapsing-remitting MS.[10] Cognitive relapse may also accompany neurological relapse.[11]

Not all cognitive parameters are equally impacted in people with MS. The most frequently impaired are processing speed and visual and verbal memory (figure 2.1).[12] Recently, researchers have addressed a key question: is there a distinct cognitive phenotype, or profile, according to disease progression? Cognitive data were collected from 1,212 people with MS seen at eight MS centers in Italy over the course of 10 years.[13] Five relatively distinct groups were detected: cognitively intact (19.4%), mild verbal memory/semantic fluency (29.9%), mild multidomain (19.5%), severe executive/attention (13.8%), and severe multidomain (17.5%) deficits, respectively. Individuals who were cognitively intact or who had mild deficits were more likely to be younger and have disease of a shorter duration, whereas the two groups with severe cognitive phenotypes were more likely to comprise people with progressive disease.

There is now abundant evidence that these deficits have a negative effect on numerous activities of daily living. Cognitively impaired people

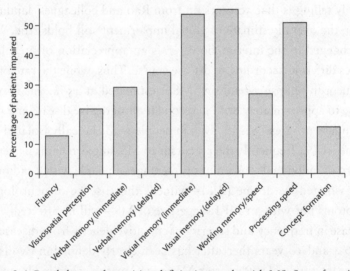

Figure 2.1. Breakdown of cognitive deficits in people with MS. See ref. 12 in chap. 2.

with MS are less likely to remain employed,[14,15] maintain relationships, and pursue leisure activities.[16] Even such basic activities as making a bed, opening containers, operating appliances, using utensils, and unshelving food become a struggle for many of those impaired.[16] The shadow cast by cognitive impairments can therefore be long and the consequences profound, as the following case histories reveal.

Let us start with information processing speed, an aspect of cognitive function that is particularly vulnerable in people with MS. Just as someone with MS may walk slower, so too thinking can slow. We live in a fast-paced world. Time hurries by and we hurry after it, chasing deadlines, locked into schedules that demand speed, efficiency, and above all, multitasking.

Susan is a 34-year-old pharmacist. Everything about her speaks to neatness, orderliness. She is a small woman, hair closely cropped, dressed in a pristine white T-shirt, crisp jeans, and spotless white sneakers. She sits forward in her chair, earnestly following what I am saying, her brow furrowed and a look of mild perplexity on her face. She has been referred to my clinic with a complaint of "memory difficulties." Detailed neuropsychological testing has, however, revealed her episodic memory to be intact, news of which is surprising to her and is the source of her perplexity. Where she had failed on testing was not in the acquisition and recall of new material but rather in the speed with which she completed tasks that demanded her attention and taxed her memory. Take away the speed component, and her performance on memory tests was good, and in some cases, better than good, or to use the adjective applied by the psychometrician, "superior," a rating that often brings a fleeting smile to the faces of people with MS when I tell them their results. What I now must impart to her is an explanation for why her faulty cognition has put an end to her blossoming career as a pharmacist. But first I need her to tell me about her work.

Susan works in a general hospital and is responsible for taking prescriptions from the physicians on both the surgical and medical floors, making up the orders, and dispensing the medications. She is one of a team of five pharmacists, and the hospital is busy, always busy she informs me. No sooner has she taken her place at the bench at 8:30 a.m. than the phone starts ringing with orders that need to be made up. Phones ring simultaneously, multiple prescriptions arrive together, some marked a higher priority than others, pagers are buzzing with the more urgent requests, and then there are the patients arriving at the counter asking for advice or to complain about something, such as why a generic drug was given instead of the brand name or why the price of a certain, essential drug has skyrocketed.

As I sit and listen to this earnest, passionate description of what her workday entails, it is soon readily apparent why she is struggling. Everything must be done quickly. Yes, one can prioritize, but even that has to be done in haste with little time for deliberation or mulling things over. This is the way general hospital pharmacies operate, as much by tradition as necessity, the apothecaries at the beck and call of imperious doctors and a demanding public. When lives are on the line, the necessity of speed is understandable, but step away from the emergency medical situation and Susan still confronts an impatient medical system that demands immediate attention and fast, efficient service. This is her undoing. Two years back she could answer a phone call from the ward while counting out 36 tablets of an antibiotic all the while signaling to a restless customer at the service counter that she would be with him in a minute. Imperceptibly, bit by bit, this had become harder to do. And remember this, she tells me, there is no room for error, not in her line of work.

Susan clearly remembers the moment when she became aware she was in trouble workwise. It had to do with the preparation of a complex intravenous solution. The patient was very ill. The nurse was badgering Susan to hurry up, but shifting into a higher gear was simply not possible. The more she tried, the more flustered she became and doubt crept in, slowing her still further. Eventually, the surgeon bellowed his frustrations down the line, bawling her out for what he perceived as tardiness, but what Susan realized in her panic was an inability to adjust her responses to the speed with which decisions were being made all around her. A colleague had stepped in and saved the day, but Susan's disability had been exposed, and while one subpar performance was not unheard of in the furious bustle of the pharmacy, when it was re-peated a week later, she was called in to the head pharmacist's office for a chat.

It turns out Susan had not disclosed her illness to her work colleagues. She chose to do so now. Everyone was sympathetic. And surprised. "Multiple sclerosis? Really? But you look so well," they told her. There was no cane. No physical signs of an illness that people often associate with a wheelchair. Ah, it must be mild then, thankfully, concluded her boss. Her poor performance over the past few weeks was put down to the undoubted stress that came with the diagnosis and living with a tough disease. Everyone in the pharmacy was very sweet, she remem-bers. She was given a couple of weeks' leave. "Why not go down to Mexico for a break, get a bit of sun, put the hurly-burly behind you, and come back refreshed?" her boss suggested. Which is what Susan and her husband did. They had a great time, and she came back deeply tanned, which offset the ivory white of the T-shirts she was so fond of. All her colleagues were glad to see her looking so well.

Two days into work, the problem recurred. Susan botched an IV, lag-ging behind the exasperated entreaties of the intensive care nurse to hurry up. When the next prescription came from the ICU, there was a little note attached asking for another pharmacist to make up the solu-tion. Susan recalls feeling devastated.

Despite her obvious struggles at work, neither Susan nor her boss put the problem down to cognitive impairment. They still assumed stress was the culprit, blaming the diagnosis of MS and its long reach. What was apparent to everyone in the pharmacy was that when the pace of work dropped, in those merciful lulls between the deluge of phone calls, beeps, and buzzers, Susan functioned like her old self. Miss Efficiency, as her colleagues called her, was back. These brief interludes, welcome as they were, proved misleading. "You see," her boss pointed out cheer-ily, "things fall apart when you are stressed. Get some help from a psychiatrist, and the problem will be solved." Everyone wanted Susan to succeed. She was popular with her colleagues and patients. The phar-macy could not slow down, so she would have to speed up. Stress re-duction was the way forward, the solution. Susan believed it too, for by now her failures at work had put her on edge, introducing a germ of uncertainty that niggled at her self-confidence, sparking waves of anxiety that were new to her, someone who had always been so controlled, in charge, super-organized. Which is how she had made her way to my clinic, the terse hastily scribbled note from her GP mentioning MS stress as the source of all her problems at work.

My clinical assessment revealed that Susan was mildly anxious but not depressed. The source of her anxiety was her work performance. When I recommended neuropsychological testing, she appeared surprised. Holding firm to her belief that stress underlay her problem, she queried how cognitive testing would help her. I didn't tell her then that the likelihood of finding impairment was as high as 45% given her relapsing-remitting disease course. That would only have made her anxiety worse and the testing more stressful. Somewhat skeptically, she went off to see the neuropsychologist.

One month later, Susan returned to my clinic for her results. She was clearly tense, on edge, and concerned about what she might hear because she found the testing process surprisingly difficult. "I think I did very badly," she confided. "I am sure I failed everything." Her eyes welled with tears. I tried to reassure her by explaining that comprehensive neuropsychological testing was not like a school examination in which one can ace all the questions and emerge with a close to perfect score. Everyone made errors. If they didn't, the world would be made up of millions of Einsteins. The recognition of this absurdity, or perhaps the mental imagery of the planet densely populated by avuncular geniuses having a bad hair day, softened her grim forebodings. A thin smile broke through the tears.

I started the feedback by informing her that prior to the onset of her multiple sclerosis she was a woman of above average intelligence. She seemed nonplussed by this observation. "How do you turn back the clock to work this out?" she wanted to know. The answer has to do with her reading skills. The ability to correctly pronounce a series of words ranging from simple, monosyllabic words—such as "plumb," "know," and "most"—to more complex, multisyllabic words—such as "hegemony," "ubiquitous," and "perspicuity"—provides an index of premorbid (pre-MS) intelligence. Learning to read is one of the first cognitive tasks we are taught and is relatively resistant to decline even in the presence of a degenerative disease like MS. This observation has led to the development of a number of reading tests that are linguistically and culturally sensitive. The Wechsler Test of Adult Reading[17] is widely used in North America. It entails the subject reading 50 words aloud and being marked according to phonetic accuracy. The resultant tally provides a marker of what a person's intellectual ability was like before the onset of illness. I should add that the testers have the phonetic spellings in front of them on the scoring sheet just in case the correct pronunciations of words like "insouciant" and "lugubrious" escape them too.

Having discussed the theory behind the reading test with Susan, I went on to tell her that there were many aspects of her cognition that remained intact. Her memory for learning new material, both verbal and visual, was good, as were her visuospatial capabilities. Executive functions (her ability to plan and problem solve and adopt flexible strategies for doing so) were intact, as were her verbal fluency and language abilities in general.

I paused in my summation and observed how she was taking the news thus far. The wan smile that had greeted news of her high pre-MS intelligence was gone and a look of perplexity was back. The good news conveyed in my opening remarks had not assuaged her anxiety, and skepticism lurked. "How can my memory be good," she challenged me, "if I can't remember how to put together the components of some of the intravenous solutions I am required to prepare?" My answer went to the heart of her limitations—namely, her impaired processing speed. "If your boss would put you in a quiet room," I told her, "and if he gave you enough time, and only one task at a time, and if he turned off the pagers and held the telephone calls, and if there was no impatient member of the general public hopping around at the customer counter clearing his throat to gain your attention, then you would get the prescription filled without error."

My answer was greeted by silence. And then a tear formed, a single tear, and it ran slowly down her cheek. "But that would be impossible,"

Susan responded softly, talking to herself as much as to me. "That is not how we work." And she is right. That is not how a busy pharmacy in a general hospital works. Her processing speed deficits had collided with the realities of the real world, and in a collision of two unequal forces, there can be only one outcome. The exigencies of her work demanded speed allied to multitasking and an ability to shut out distractions in the moment. When speed of processing slows, things start falling apart. The ability to think quickly, to put sequences together quickly, to respond quickly, and to link these lightning responses to accuracy are all non-negotiable. These are the basic building blocks of Susan's job, and central to it all, the hub around which everything else rotates, is her speed of processing information. Now it has been compromised, fatally so, and despite her many other abilities and strengths, despite a sympathetic boss and understanding colleagues, and most painful of all, despite a lifetime of high achievement in which she met and conquered all her challenges, this current hurdle is too great. There are no accommodations that she can be given, no quiet room on offer; no one can slow the clocks, turn off the phones, or make the public more patient. There is no slack in the system to carry a team player who is underperforming. Susan was 34 years old and her career as a hospital pharmacist was over. Other options, however, were still open to her. Six weeks of computerized cognitive rehabilitation led to a modest increase in processing speed and with it the door opened to a quieter dispensary far removed from the organized mayhem of a general hospital. But how she missed her former life. She had thrived on the buzz of it all, the fast-paced challenge of cutting-edge therapeutics, replaced now by salves, emollients, evacuants, expectorants, and soporifics—no less important to those who needed them, she is quick to point out, but by comparison, oh so mundane.

There are a number of ways that processing speed can be tested. The one favored by neuropsychologists who assess people with MS is the Symbol Digit Modalities Test (SDMT).[18] In the conventional administration of the test, the person with MS is handed a piece of paper which contains a code listing nine symbols matched to nine numbers (figure 2.2).

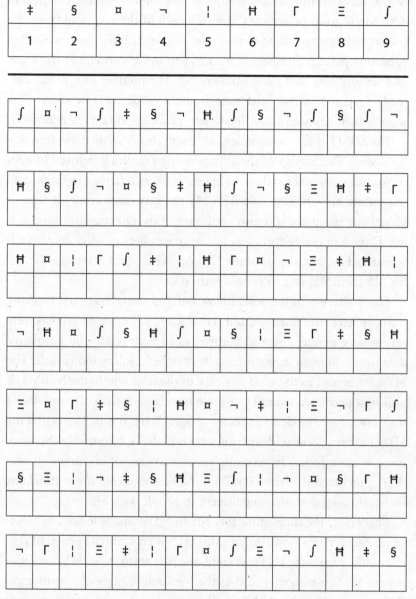

Figure 2.2. Example of stimuli of the Symbol Digit Modalities Test (SDMT) type. See ref. 34 in chap. 2.

Below this two-line code are rows of the same symbols. The person with MS is given 90 seconds to match each of these symbols with the correct number according to the code. The oral rather than the written version is preferred in people with MS to bypass arm/hand weakness and sensory loss that slow handwriting. The number of symbols correctly matched in this brief time frame provide the raw score. This score is then adjusted according to age, gender, and years of education.

The SDMT is easy to complete, although clearly more difficult to perform well. The brevity of the administration makes it beloved of neuropsychologists and psychometricians, while its relative simplicity does not induce anxiety in people with MS the way more complex tests of processing speed do. It is also predictive of overall cognitive functioning. Data supporting this comes from researchers in Belgium who administered the test as part of the Neuropsychological Screening Battery for MS (NSBMS) to 359 people with MS.[19]

This battery also has tests for verbal and visual memory, working memory, executive function, and verbal fluency. Various thresholds were set for determining global cognitive impairment relative to normative data obtained from demographically matched healthy individuals. The SDMT emerged as the most sensitive of the tests within the NSBMS. It also best predicted overall cognitive impairment with a sensitivity of 0.91 but a more modest specificity of 0.60. What this tells us is that the SDMT is very good at identifying who is globally, cognitively impaired, but it is less effective in detecting those who are *not* impaired. The authors concluded that the SDMT should be considered *the* sentinel test in determining cognitive impairment in people with MS.

There is strong support for this opinion. The Multiple Sclerosis Outcome Assessments Consortium (MSOAC) is an umbrella group of representatives from the US Food and Drug Administration (FDA), the European Medicines Agency (EMA), the National Institute of Neurological Disorders and Stroke (NINDS), pharmaceutical companies, advocacy groups, academic institutions, and people with MS. One of their aims is to ascertain performance outcomes that are valid, reliable, cost effective, practical, and relevant to those with MS. The SDMT has been deemed to meet all these criteria. Additional strengths were noted to include excellent psychometrics, brevity, low cost, patient friendliness, easy translatability, and its availability by computer administration. Most importantly, the test is considered a good marker for change over time that is clinically meaningful. The threshold decided upon here is four points, commensurate with a 10% shift in performance.[20] Finally, there are well-replicated MS-specific imaging data that confirm the utility of the SDMT as a pivotal cognitive measure both clinically and from a research perspective. It correlates more robustly than any other cognitive measure with numerous brain MRI metrics in people with MS. These associations are stronger for measures of atrophy—such as third ventricle width (a marker for thalamic atrophy)[21,22] and neocortical atrophy[23]—than lesion volume.[21] These structural findings are complemented by an understanding of the functional neuroanatomy of the SDMT in healthy people[24] and, by comparison, the reduced bilateral frontoparietal and ancillary insula, thalamic, and anterior cingulate activations seen in people with MS.[25]

With the stamp of approval from the MSOAC, it is not surprising that the SDMT is now regarded as a valid clinical trial endpoint for measuring cognition in people with MS.[26] In this regard, it has replaced the Paced Auditory Serial Addition Test (PASAT),[27] for many years the standard bearer of processing speed determination. Originally devised to test people with traumatic brain injury, the PASAT entails the aural presentation of a series of digits from one to nine. Participants are instructed to add each new digit to the one that preceded it. Part of the challenge lies in giving the tester the correct total, while at the same time remembering the last digit to add to the next one (figure 2.3). The speed at which the digits are given varies. By tradition, the most frequently used intervals are two and three seconds. In general, the faster the presentation, the greater number of the errors made.[28]

In a longitudinal study over one year, the SDMT was found to be slightly superior to the three-second PASAT in predicting overall cognitive dysfunction.[29] More important, the SDMT was completed by all subjects and healthy control subjects, whereas corresponding percentages for the PASAT-3 were 86.9% and 94.7%, respectively, attesting to the latter test's greater difficulty, and by extension, anxiety-inducing tendencies.

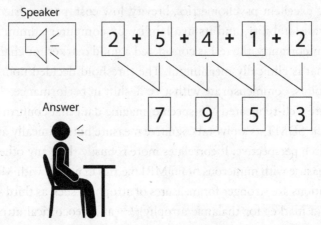

Figure 2.3. The aural version of the Paced Auditory Serial Addition Test (PASAT)

A similar preference emerged from an analysis of data from 14 MS disease-modifying registration trials where the SDMT consistently outperformed the PASAT-3, which led the authors to endorse the SDMT as the measure of choice in MS trials assessing processing speed.[26]

Having firmly supplanted the PASAT as the measure of choice in assessing processing speed, the SDMT is now also considered the single best psychometric test for people with MS across all cognitive domains. There is a general recognition that, in a busy neurological practice, time and the absence of neuropsychological expertise preclude not only a detailed neuropsychological assessment but also briefer screening measures that encompass multiple cognitive domains. In a situation like this, the National MS Society (NMSS) in the United States, the Consortium of Multiple Sclerosis Centers (CMSC), and the International Multiple Sclerosis Cognition Society (IMSCOGS) all endorse the SDMT as their measure of choice. Their collective recommendations include utilizing the test for early baseline testing when the person with MS is clinically stable and, at a minimum, repeating it annually, or more often if clinically indicated.[30]

Time and again I am witness in my clinic to how slowed processing speed can bring someone down. The man sitting ill at ease before me is a natty dresser. Everything about him is stylish—his chiseled build, the trim cut of his clothes, a racy hairstyle, the shades that peek out from his blazer's breast pocket, the slim, supple leather folio case that rests on his lap, the latest model iPhone in a matching leather case clipped on to the side of the attaché, and the fine Italian shoes beautifully polished that come to a point. All the clothes, accessories, and accruements color coordinated. He is simply one cool man, in touch with the fashion and zeitgeist of his times, riding a wave of contemporary, chic, smooth elegance.

Or, rather, he was. The journey has come to an end. The appearance, however, endures. MS has deprived him of much, but it cannot, *will not*, he asserts, remove his persona, the outward display of a man once confident and at the top of his game. Roger is 44 years of age and until six months ago held a senior position in a multinational advertising agency. He described his job to me, and it certainly sounded appealing. He would be approached by a client who invariably had very deep pockets. A high-end product needed exposure—global exposure but pitched at that rarefied level that set it apart from competitors. This drive for exclusivity went hand in hand with money, lots of it, which meant that the advertising campaign to be developed came with a large budget too, no need to skimp in getting the creative juices flowing. With an open checkbook in front of him, Roger's ideas more often than not drifted to glamorous locales, far away islands, alluring cities like Venice and Barcelona, remote communities that survive in extreme environments like the Sahel or Antarctic—places that seize the imagination of the audiences who would view the finished product with a mix of wanderlust, yearning, and a tacit recognition that there was another world out there, the mythical 1%, the super-affluent, oh so desirable but unattainable. But who is to stop a person dreaming? And so, these skilled advertisers, these dream merchants, go about their magic, creating a charmed world that appears on giant billboards, in two-minute video pop-ups that intrude into your morning reading of your online newspaper, stopping viewers in their tracks, a welcome momentary pause in a busy, harried life. Just for a moment, there appears the vision of something wonderfully different, the glimpse of which sends people hurrying off to buy a piece of it, a small token of an existence that could never be lived other than in that fleeting moment.

What a world this chic, smart, and trendy man created. This arbiter of taste and refinement rode his profession hard for 10 years, a decade at the top, flying business class to the four corners of the world. I had a sense that if Elon Musk established his outpost on Mars, Roger would have been given the gig to sell the planet to weary earthlings hungry for change and a shot in the arm. It had been a great decade, he reminisced. So many interesting people met, places visited, experiences savored. When his MS first presented, it hardly slowed him down. A spot of visual trouble, followed by some transitory weakness. To be sure, the diagnosis was a shock. He remembers receiving it one bitterly cold Toronto morning. The snow was falling thickly, the temperatures had plummeted, an ice storm was on the way, and he was in a hurry to get to the airport to catch a flight to the French Caribbean. And now this graying physician, kindly and unhurried in his demeanor and speech, was telling him that his nervous system was faulty, that the sheaths enveloping his neurons had become inflamed and that was why his thigh felt numb and his visual field on the left was blurry. MS. Two little letters with the power of an A-bomb. "It can't be," Roger recalled thinking. "Not me. Not now." There was a plane to catch. Somewhere warm was waiting with white sands and turquoise waters and swaying palms. He was running late. He would miss his flight. He thanked the neurologist, fled his office, flung himself into the waiting limo, and buried what he had just been told. MS, or what he knew of the disease, did not sit well with a jet-setting lifestyle and a profession that lionized perfection, fantasy, and limitless possibilities.

Avoidance is not a good coping strategy. We will return to this later. But for now, let us stay with the advertising executive hurrying toward the departure lounge at Pearson International Airport. I have until now confined my description to his appearance. I put it first because it was so striking, so perfectly in tune with his world and what he created. Appearances, however, soon fade. A smart suit will not hold a psychiatrist's attention. Personality, on the other hand, will. And Roger's appearance and personality moved in tandem, a happy marriage, the exterior elegance at one with a keen, sharp, and perceptive mind; moreover, a mind that was empathic and sensitive to those around him. The jet-set existence had not disconnected him from the world of the other 99%, the bustle of life on a treadmill, where if you fell off, it was hard to get back on again. He knew this difficulty all too well because he had been there once, and after tasting it you never forgot it. Success had not made him arrogant. Rather, it had left him feeling grateful, thankful for his good fortune and the opportunity to live life on his own terms. This mix of elegance with honest, perceptive insight was beguiling. Spend a little time in Roger's company and you felt good. If he made me, his psychiatrist, feel this way—what in the jargon of my profession is referred to as a positive countertransference—then his clients would surely have felt the same way too. It was easy to see why he had been so successful in his professional and personal life. And then MS intruded.

Eight years into his disease, fatigue had become something of a problem. Roger worked around this, learning to delegate, taking 10-minute power naps, and boosting his flagging energy with long-acting methylphenidate (Ritalin) tablets. The part he could not camouflage, skirt, or offload, however, was his increasing cognitive dysfunction. He moved in a fast-paced world. Decisions flowed through him, and he had a large team to manage. Group meetings were proving increasingly tough to negotiate. He prided himself of his choice of staff—young, smart, quick-witted creative people. This is what drove advertising. All these razor-sharp intellects in one open-concept office, their energies feeding off one another, ideas batted around at high speed, picked up, discarded, and recycled, the incessant chatter of high-energy, productive individuals creating a concept that could influence millions of people. Yes, "millions" is correct. That's the market out there, great swathes of society in thrall to the gurus of Madison Avenue. But what once had been his favorite preserve, the company's sleek state-of-the-art boardroom, had now become his greatest source of stress and anxiety. He had loved the group energy that permeated the room when it was filled with his team—the intensity of the moment when ideas that had started as mere abstractions coalesced into something more tangible, reality taking shape before them all, given momentum, legs, and most fun of all, a name, the corporate signature melded to the emotive music that was either lifted from Mozart or Pink Floyd or commissioned. There it was on the big screen, two minutes of distilled magic, the product of so much time and distance and attention—myriad details, none too small, playing out against the backdrop of the golden buildings of Nouakchott as a blazing African sun set and the ouds and violins tugged at the heartstrings. Who could resist this? It gave them all a high. And best of all, it showed them the future too, for success bred success and no sooner had the sun set in Mauritania than it rose in the East, and the next project beckoned.

Roger recalled the day it all started to unravel. The process had been gradual, he could see this now in retrospect, but pushing away concerns, blotting his mind to the reality taking form within, was now no longer sustainable. The meeting had adjourned. Another successful project was behind his team, but a few of his closest associates had noticed that he appeared out of sorts. A little slow on the uptake, slightly hesitant in his responses, left behind momentarily as the high-speed train of creativity rushed around the room pinging from person to person. Slumped in his private office after the meeting broke up, Roger felt none of the usual post-project rush, the high that always signaled another inspired creation. He had made his excuses, opting out of the traditional decamping to the wine bar down the road where a successful product launch was always celebrated with overflowing glasses of Moët & Chandon, which by the way was another of his satisfied corporate clients.

Euphoria had given way to worry. Roger conceded that at times he had felt adrift during the team meeting. He could not keep up with the banter and exchange of ideas. He had lost the thread of what was taking place, and no sooner had he caught up in one of the momentary lulls that came with a coffee break than he lost the plot again. There were only so many deferrals he could make, only so many waves of the hand gesturing to someone else for an opinion when all eyes were really on him, waiting for his critique or praise. Most embarrassing of all, when the presentation ended and his entire team looked to him for his imprimatur, he had missed his cue. He was still a couple of steps behind, desperately trying to play catch-up, wondering what the next steps would be even when there were none—all that was left was just a thumbs up to give to his team, and a big bravo to sign off on the project. The finality of the moment only dawned on him when he became aware of the silence in the room and the bemused looks on the faces of his staff. To cover his lapse, he feigned feeling overwhelmed by what he had just seen, and his team bought it, their relief manifest. Alone now with his troubled thoughts he could see with clarion certainty that he had indeed been overwhelmed, but for a very different reason. He thought he was losing his mind.

I went through Roger's cognitive results with him test by test. Attention was borderline normal. Episodic memory remained intact. Language had been spared. Visual-spatial abilities were robust. Problem solving skills fell in the normal range. The one cognitive piece that was missing was intact processing speed. It had slowed to the point where running a top-notch advertising team had become an insurmountable challenge. Again, we come back to the importance of speed—there was no place in the cut-throat world of advertising for slowness. Nothing moved at a pedestrian place here, least of all ideas and the energy that gave them life. Everything zipped along, top gear all the way, no place for laggards, slow pokes, or stodginess. Speed was prized, part of the attraction of the job, this symbiosis of new ideas and the ability to run with them quickly. Slow things down and the works gummed up. Sluggish was not a word synonymous with Roger's profession. But that was how he felt. Sluggish. What an awful word, with all its unfortunate connotations. It hobbled his creativity. Add even a tincture of it to his world and creativity floundered.

Accommodations were not an option. Not in the one-dimensional world of fast, faster, and fastest. He was the fulcrum around which his team moved. He had to problem solve, quickly. He needed to make executive decisions, quickly. He had to access his own fund of knowledge and accumulated wisdom, quickly. People were in and out of his office all day long with their problems, new ideas, solutions, queries. They even moved quickly, in step with their thoughts. No time to say, "Whoa! Give me a moment." A truth that had been present for years, pushing its way ever more insistently to the surface only to be chased away resolutely, could no longer be ignored. Work, a source of great joy and intellectual nourishment, a place of conviviality and camaraderie, a marker of where

Roger stood in this world, and a testimony to his intellect, success, and personal acumen, had been slipping away from him for nearly two years. Imperceptibly, the tasks he was called on to do had become harder. He could see it now and was painfully aware of the lengths he had gone to in order to keep himself afloat. The longer hours spent at the office. The weekends devoted to work instead of socializing. The multiple sticky notes that plastered his desk at work and his fridge at home. The endless to-do lists that took up pages in his organizer. The one-on-one meetings that he now preferred instead of group contacts because he found it easier when there was only one person talking rather than many. It had all fallen apart because of poor information processing speed. His finely tuned aesthetic sensibilities were still there, but he had lost the ability to manage a complex, thoroughbred stable of likeminded intellects.

Extraordinary abilities had allowed him to hide his escalating deficits this far. Had he worked in a different field, perhaps this day of reckoning could have been pushed down the road a little more. But not in the unforgiving world of niche advertising. Compassion was not a guiding principle when there was so much money at stake and so little margin to get things wrong. The contrasts were stark. You either performed or you failed. You were either successful or you were not. You either delivered or you didn't. No shades of gray here, and now the balance had tipped irrevocably downward. A disability plan awaited.

Where do you go in life when fate has played a cruel hand? What is it like to scale the heights of the advertising world, start a fad, sway a demographic, and see the far-flung corners of the world, with all its wonders, through the most fortunate, privileged, and comfortable of lenses, only to have it taken away from you when you are in your prime, a 40th birthday still a recent memory? There are no other jobs waiting. The high-wire, exhilarating ride is over, and there is no substitute. Now you face days of deep loneliness. How do you fill in the time? Your mind drifts back to the office. What is going on there today, he wonders? The thought of what he is missing torments him. Sitting at home in his comfy den, Roger knows that his former colleagues are on the go go go, putting together another package of clever ideas, with locales being excitedly scouted, flights booked, hotels arranged, and bags hurriedly packed.

And here he is alone with his memories while all around him life flows on with opportunities now tantalizingly just out of reach. It comes as no surprise to find that depression is a short hop away.

The two case histories provided thus far illustrate the pivotal role played by processing speed in determining a person's ability to function. Furthermore, there is a view that processing speed may also underpin other aspects of cognition, so that when it falters, deficits may arise in the ability to learn and consolidate new material.[31] I will expand on this theory in chapters to come, but for now let us stay with the SDMT as the sentinel maker of the quintessential cognitive failing in people with MS—namely, impaired processing speed.

The SDMT is the only test that features in all three of the most widely used and recommended cognitive batteries for people with MS. The first of these is an offshoot of a study by Rao et al.[2] that heralded the importance of cognitive dysfunction in people with MS. The Brief Repeatable Neuropsychological Battery (BRNB)[32] contains four additional cognitive tests, which probe verbal and visual memory, working memory and processing speed, verbal fluency, and executive function. The "brief" descriptor meant this screening battery could generally be completed in 40 minutes or less. The need for a more comprehensive assessment comprising tests considered sensitive to deficits typically seen in people with MS spawned the development of the Minimal Assessment of Cognitive Function in MS (MACFIMS).[33] This expanded on the BRNB by keeping some of the tests, jettisoning others, and adding new indices, thereby increasing the administration time to 90 minutes or more depending on the person being tested. The third widely used battery harkens back to a persistent clinical need for a quick, reliable, and sensitive measure of cognition in people with MS. The Brief International Cognitive Assessment in MS (BICAMS)[34] contains three of the MACFIMS tests and takes around 10 minutes to complete. It has been widely translated, making it truly an international screening battery. Details of these three batteries can be seen in table 2.1.

With the SDMT now occupying center stage as the test of choice when it comes to processing speed, a closer look at this test is required.

Table 2.1. Summary of the three most widely used and recommended cognitive batteries for multiple sclerosis

Cognitive Index	BRNB	MACFIMS	BICAMS
Learning and memory	Consistent Long-Term Retrieval Test from the Buschke Selective Reminding Test	California Verbal Learning Test	California Verbal Learning Test
	10/36 Spatial Recall Test	Brief Visuospatial Memory Test–Revised	Brief Visuospatial Memory Test–Revised
Processing speed	Symbol Digit Modalities Test (SDMT)	Symbol Digit Modalities Test (SDMT)	Symbol Digit Modalities Test (SDMT)
	Paced Auditory Serial Addition Test (3 seconds) (PASAT-3)	Paced Auditory Serial Addition Test (3 seconds) (PASAT-3)	
	Paced Auditory Serial Addition Test (2 seconds) (PASAT-2)	Paced Auditory Serial Addition Test (2 seconds) (PASAT-2)	
Executive function	Controlled Oral Word Association Test (COWAT)	Controlled Oral Word Association Test (COWAT)	
		Delis-Kaplan Executive Function System (D-KEFS)	
Verbal fluency/language	Controlled Oral Word Association Test (COWAT)	Controlled Oral Word Association Test (COWAT)	
Visual perceptions/spatial processing		Judgment of Line Orientation Test	
Duration	~40 minutes	~90 minutes	~10 minutes

Notes: BRNB = Brief Repeatable Neuropsychological Battery; MACFIMS = Minimal Assessment of Cognitive Function in M BICAMS = Brief International Cognitive Assessment in MS.

To begin with, there are a couple of drawbacks to the test which will preclude its administration in a small number of people with MS. As noted earlier, the SDMT is generally completed orally, rather than having participants write their responses. In this way, people with MS who have marked motor involvement, such as weakness of the hands or a pronounced tremor from cerebellar involvement, can complete the test without having their performance confounded by these factors. However, cerebellar involvement can also lead to a dysarthria in which speech slows and becomes slurred, and this too can increase the time taken to complete the SDMT.[35] It is, however, important to remember that while speech may slow for neurological reasons alone, impaired processing speed may impede it too.[36]

A second physical impediment to the SDMT and other visually based tests is reduced visual acuity.[37] This point is given added weight by the fact that up to 80% of people with MS can show evidence of visual impairment.[38] It is therefore a requirement that before a person with MS proceeds with testing, their visual acuity be assessed and found to be at least 20/70 binocularly.

There is another factor relating to the visual system that may contribute to a slower performance on visually presented tests like the SDMT. I refer to eye movement. When interpreting the eye movement metrics in people with MS, it is helpful to divide them into two broad categories. The first may arise in response to pathological changes in the cranial nerves, brain stem, and cerebellar circuits that control eye movement. Remember the features of Charcot's MS triad? One element is nystagmus, which refers to repetitive, uncontrollable eye movements that can occur from side to side (horizontal nystagmus), up and down (vertical nystagmus), or in a circular fashion, all of which can reduce vision. These eye movements are discernable during the neurological examination. The second category refers to subtler movement, such as a saccade, that require eye-tracking devices to detect. *Saccade*, translated from the French, means "jerky" and refers to the rapid, jerky movements of both eyes between two or more points of fixation. These are under cognitive control. Attention, working memory, and decision making, which is part of executive functioning, can all influence the saccadic network. A multifocal disease like MS is well placed to disrupt the synchronization of widely dispersed neural circuits that link ocular centers in frontal regions, such as the frontal eye fields, supplementary frontal eye fields, dorsolateral prefrontal cortex, and anterior cingulate cortex, with those in the posterior parietal cortex. While there is a substantial literature devoted to eye movement abnormalities in general in persons with MS[39–41] and links established with cognitive dysfunction,[42,43] reported associations with impairments on the SDMT are equivocal.[44–46] To further our understanding of why people with MS find the SDMT so challenging, my research team enrolled 33 people between the ages of 18 and 60 years with a confirmed diagnosis of MS and 25 demographically matched healthy people and monitored their subtle eye movements while they competed the test.[47]

The eye-tracking data were collected using the Gazepoint GP3 HD eye tracker attached to a desktop computer. The SDMT was displayed in its original form and scale on a 19-inch monitor. As with the paper version of the SDMT, the test was presented for 90 seconds and responses were recorded orally.

For the purposes of eye tracking, the SDMT was divided into two rectangular areas of interest; namely, the *key* and the *test* areas. The key area referred to the two rows of boxes, one filled with numbers 1 to 9 and the other with the nine symbols linked to each number. The test area referred to the page containing rows of symbols that must be matched to the correct number according to the key (see figure 2.2). Eye-tracking measurements included, among others, the total number of fixations (defined as maintaining visual gaze on a single location) in the test and key areas, the average fixation time in the test and key areas, the total number of visits (i.e., eye movements) to the key area, the total number of visits to the key area per response (response here refers to the attempt to match the symbol with the digit), and the mean saccade velocity.

As expected, the MS group performed significantly slower on the SDMT. What differentiated their eye-tracking responses from those in healthy individuals were the total number of visits to the key area per response and an increase in the total number of fixations in the test area. These findings expose the uncertainties and delays that characterize the performances of people with MS when given the relatively simple task of matching a number and symbol at speed. The mechanistic underpinnings to these disordered responses reflect the key role played by attention in controlling eye movements, with the secondary cognitive effects manifesting as delayed information processing speed.

Abnormal eye movement and speech are two neurological symptoms that can affect performance on the SDMT. There is also evidence, somewhat more equivocal, that shows psychiatric factors having an influence too. In a retrospective chart review of 128 people with MS, depression more than anxiety was found to have a negative influence on SDMT performance and the ability to work.[48] A differential effect on cognition between depression and anxiety also emerged in a study of 185 recently diagnosed MS individuals.[49] Lower levels of depression were associated with better attention/processing speed, whereas less anxiety was linked to better nonverbal memory performance. These findings remained unchanged after controlling for MRI-discernable lesion burden and fatigue.

The cognitively deleterious effects of depression and anxiety are not just confined to people with MS. Evidence for this emerged in a study of three immune-mediated diseases—namely, MS, inflammatory bowel disease, and rheumatoid arthritis—and of people with anxiety and depression who had no overt immune-mediated condition.[50] All four groups were found to have greater cognitive compromise in processing speed (as measured by the SDMT), verbal learning, and delayed recall relative to healthy population normative data. While depression was found to slow processing speed, the cognitive effects of anxiety were more widespread, negatively affecting not only processing speed but also verbal learning and working memory.

The literature on psychiatric factors influencing processing speed and cognition in general in people with MS is a small one. I have highlighted the positive studies here. Others studies have reached different conclusions,[51–53] so more work is needed to clarify the picture. However, should a putative association, possibly causal, be confirmed, then it potentially opens up a therapeutic avenue to boost cognition because depression and anxiety are treatable. By extension, reducing depression and anxiety may therefore have cognitive benefits too, including an improvement in processing speed. Here, studies in other disorders offer some hope. For example, in an eight-week open-label placebo-controlled trial, sertraline, a selective serotonin reuptake inhibitor, was used to successfully treat depression in people with a mild traumatic brain injury.[54] An additional benefit was that certain cognitive indices, such as short-term verbal and visual memory, psychomotor speed, and overall cognitive efficiency, improved too. These improvements were clearly linked to the effects of sertraline and not to spontaneous recovery with time. Similar evidence has emerged in people with depression who do not have a neurological illness,[55] with cognitive improvement also translating into real-world benefits; namely, improved long-term psychosocial functioning.[56]

I mentioned earlier a potential association between impaired processing speed and deficits in learning new material.[31] With this in mind, let me describe a study from my lab that dissected the components of the SDMT in search of cognitive processes other than processing speed that might come into play when a person takes the test. While most individuals complete the test by rapidly moving their eyes from the rows of symbols to the code at the top of the page and back again, the possibility of some people remembering the symbol-digit pair as they progressed through the test needs to be considered too. To address this possibility, we developed a computerized analog of the test.[57] The symbol-digit code was left untouched, but rather than present all the symbols below the code, we limited them to a single line only (figure 2.4). Unlike the conventional SDMT, which you will remember records the number of correct symbol-number matches in 90 seconds, the computerized analog records the time taken to complete each line.

Subjects still have to match the symbols to the numbers as quickly as possible, just as they are required to do in the original test, but as they complete the last symbol-number pairing, the line of symbols is replaced by another. At exactly the same time, the symbol-number code, which is fixed in the traditional test described above, changes too. The person completing the test is not warned of it and indeed will not be aware of the change (unless, and this is highly unlikely, the person has

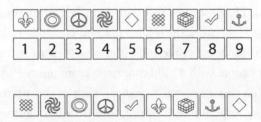

Figure 2.4. Computerized analog of the SDMT

instantly memorized the original coding). By changing the code each time a new line of symbols appears (this takes place eight times), we have effectively removed any memory component from the SDMT.

Having devised this computerized memory-free variant of the SDMT, we set about comparing it to a computerized version in which the code remains fixed throughout the sequential appearance of the eight lines of symbols. The two tests are therefore identical, save for one characteristic—the fixity or otherwise of the symbol-digit code. We administered each version of the test to two groups of 50 people with MS and 33 healthy participants. The results are shown in figures 2.5A and B.

Let's start with the healthy subjects, those whose performance is shown in figure 2.5A. What is readily apparent is that performance speeds up in the fixed trial, as indicated by the downward slope of the regression line shown in black circles. Why should this be? Well, there are two likely explanations. The first is that the subjects become increasingly familiar with the test as it proceeds, thereby making it easier—essentially faster—to complete. This improvement is indicative of practice effects. The second explanation is that as the test proceeds, some subjects begin memorizing the symbol-digit code and no longer have to move their eyes to and from the code, which can also speed up performance.

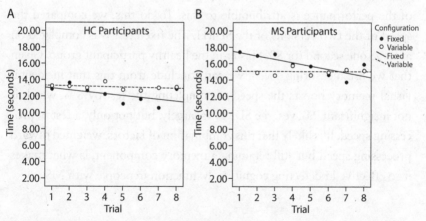

Figure 2.5. Performance on a computerized SDMT analog in healthy control (HC) participants (*A*) and people with MS (*B*) across eight trials comparing the fixed versus variable configurations

Let's now look at the test in which the symbol-digit code changes. Here, performance in the healthy participants is shown in the dotted line with white circles. The speed of performance over the course of the eight trials does not get faster. The line essentially remains flat. This group will also have become increasingly familiar with the test as it proceeded through eight trials, just as in the group above. But familiarity alone did not speed up performance. From this we can conclude that the increase in speed over time in the fixed-code version of the test is attributable to memory, or to be more precise, a particular kind of memory, incidental visual memory. "Incidental" refers here to the fact that subjects were not asked to memorize anything—the learning or memory component was generated incidentally or automatically.

If we now look at the results for the MS group, we see exactly the same phenomenon. Those given the fixed-code test (*black dots*) get faster over the eight trials, whereas those completing the variable version (*white dots*) do not. The only difference between people with MS and healthy subjects is that the MS group does both tests a lot slower, but we could have predicted this beforehand, for as the histories described earlier show, slowed processing speed is a hallmark cognitive failing in people with MS.

Having established that the SDMT does indeed contain an incidental visual memory component, the last question we addressed was how much of the performance is attributable to this. To do this, we compared the speed of the two versions of the SDMT. The fixed test was completed on average one second (or 8%) faster in the healthy participant group. Given that we are measuring speed, we can conclude from this that incidental visual memory boosts the speed of completing the test by 8%, which is not insignificant. So, yes, the SDMT is largely, but not only, a test of processing speed. It is likely that this combination of factors, weighted toward processing speed but still retaining a memory component, is what makes it so effective in detecting cognitive dysfunction in people with MS.

[THREE]

More on Processing Speed and the Tyranny of Distraction

WHEN PROCESSING SPEED slows, it does not only affect people in high-end jobs. Step back from the dizzying heights of Madison Avenue, or the life-and-death prescriptions that must be filled without delay, and enter a more familiar world, one inhabited by millions of employees each day. I refer to the administrative assistant's office. Here, the décor is simple, practical, cost effective. A sturdy desk, on which sits a plastic in-out tray and a framed photograph of a spouse with two teenage kids, a computer workstation attached to a printer, a chair that is not ergonomically friendly, a hulking metal filing cabinet, and propped up in the corner, a plastic floral arrangement beneath a framed motivational print, the one concession to aesthetics in an otherwise utilitarian space.

Felicity sits in front of the computer screen; she is a loving wife and the proud mom to the two gangly teenagers in the photo, with their toothy grins advertising the orthodontist's handiwork. She has had multiple sclerosis for 15 years and walks with a slight limp, one leg being weaker than the other. She has resisted using a cane—"The mark of Cain," she bitingly refers to it—because she believes her job is under threat. The company has recently downsized and 10% of the staff were euphemistically "let go." "Fired" is how she views it, and she sees herself next in line if she brings attention to her disability. "Who will give a middle-aged woman with MS a job?" she asks me rhetorically. "I have been with the company 20 years. Straight out of college and into the same office I have now. The furniture may have changed over the years and the computers upgraded," she laughs, "but two things have remained constant, me and the plastic flowers." And, of the two, it must be said that the artificial blooms are faring better. For what brings her to my office is a concern that she has had for a year or so. She cannot keep up with her boss. Same boss, same workload, subpar performance. She tearfully produces her annual work performance appraisal. She has never received one like it before. Words like "inefficient" and "sloppy" jump off the page, a whole new lexicon unfamiliar to her. She places a review from five years back alongside the latest one and the contrast is immediately apparent. Felicity is failing at work.

I start by acknowledging her concerns. She has given her working life to one organization. She has done her nine-to-five bit, a real trooper, never late or slipping away early, stepping up when overtime has been needed, typing her boss's reports, getting him his early afternoon coffee, watching his children grow up alongside hers in a parallel universe, never resenting their private schools, swimming pool, expensive holidays, and Ivy League frat houses. When her MS first presented with limb weakness, she took two weeks' sick leave and then picked up where she had left off. Felicity never even claimed the sick days, choosing to chalk up her absence to vacation time because rumor had it the company was in a little trouble and the chop was coming for some. Her pay was modest but considered fair market value for what she did. Her benefits package was excellent. She could not afford the $25,000 disease-modifying drug that she took daily without it. When she added her salary to her husband's pay, they got by as a family and could afford the metal work that would in time given their children beautiful smiles. Now, her hard won lifestyle was under threat, undermined by her MS. Her fears were easily understood.

I asked Felicity to describe her workday to me. "The phones start ringing before I even get in," she told me. "Phones?" I queried. "More than one?" It turns out there were two, one for the company at large and then the boss's private line for family, friends, and select clients, 50 or so individuals whose business accounted for more than half the company's profits. "It's a good thing I have two ears," she divulged with a bright smile. But her eyes gave her away—there was no mirth in her quip.

Two telephones, one on each ear, would challenge anyone's attention, let alone someone whose cognition is faltering. What Felicity was being asked to do was at times akin to a dichotic listening task, a particular cognitive challenge in which an individual is subject to simultaneous but different auditory streams of information, one channeled into the left ear and the other into the right. The task probes the efficiency with which the two hemispheres of the brain communicate with one another and is dependent on the functional integrity of that broad band of white matter fibers, the corpus callosum, that links the right and left sides of the brain. This great mass of white matter is susceptible to demyelination, one of the core pathological processes in MS. An MRI can show this clearly, with a distinctive pattern of shrinkage or atrophy of the fibers accompanied at times by lesions that show up either dark or light depending on the scan sequence. As Felicity spoke, I had her MRI images up before me, and that distinctive punched-out pattern of lesions within the corpus callosum was clearly visible.

Felicity's work was much more than answering telephones. She had to type reports, take down memoranda, use shorthand to capture verbatim what her boss wanted typed, manage both of their electronic diaries, liaise with other staff including secretarial colleagues in the other backroom offices, make lunch reservations for business meetings, attend to menus while catering for special food requests and allergies, settle certain accounts, maintain the petty cash box, send and receive faxes (remember those, Doc?), scan documents, file a mountain of paperwork, recycle what was not needed, empty the recycle and trash bins, order the office stationery, make sure the toners didn't run dry, and keep the pencils sharpened, all the while ensuring her desk remained neat and tidy, everything in the proper place, orderly and efficient because, remember this, she was the face of a company that distributed health care products, the first person new clients saw when they entered the office, and the impression she made, notwithstanding the ersatz flowers and the cheesy wall slogan exhorting team spirit, went a long way. Oh, and one other thing! Occasionally, she had to do her boss a special favor, such as contacting his family doctor for a repeat prescription of his anti-hypertensive medications, or booking the airport limo for his wife, or sorting out the babysitter for the evening (but that's going back years), and once, just once, picking up his laundry. Felicity paused in her check-list, mulling over what she had just told me, a look of mild surprise intermingled with wonder settling over her features as if for the first time becoming fully aware of just how much she had been asked to do.

There is a coda to all of this that is the clincher from an MS-cognitive perspective. Everything, absolutely everything, has to be done quickly. Top speed, foot off the brake, time is money, because remember the company has been struggling a little of late, a downturn in the economy demanding they all crank up the speed still further, every last drop of efficiency squeezed from a shrinking work pool. A year back, Felicity's myelin was healthier. She could multitask because her processing speed was intact. But imperceptibly it had slipped, and now, no matter how hard she tried, drawing on her vast well of experience and super orga-nizational skills, digging deep into an intact repository of memory that had stood her in such good stead for 20 years in that front office, she had exhausted her compensatory skills. The way she saw it, the lemon had been squeezed dry.

There is no flexibility in the system for people whose cognition has slowed. Think of Formula 1 or NASCAR. There are no kudos for get-ting around the circuit without crashing your car if you drive slowly. But there will be no kudos either if you drive too fast and crash. The great challenge here is to marry speed and accuracy. It's a perennial chal-lenge nearly all of us face in our working lives. The perfect balance is to find that sweet spot where both attributes are optimized. Tilt too far toward speed and the wheels fall off. Lean a little too far in the other direction and the moment is lost. It's something that cognitive scientists must account for when assessing neuropsychological performance. When we give a person a test of processing speed, we need to keep an eye on accuracy too. My patient, the loyal, experienced, and hardwork-ing administrative assistant, had not initially been aware of this tradeoff when, in response to the admonishments of her boss and coworkers to please hurry up, she started to make mistake after mistake. Her errors were pointed out to her, patiently to begin with but with increasing impatience as she appeared unable to right the ship of her failing intellect. The harder she pushed to keep on time with her tasks, the more mistakes popped up. Juggling her numerous tasks proved increasingly difficult. Two years back, Felicity could keep three or four balls in the air at any one time as she blitzed through the day. Now answering the phone while typing a document proved discombobulating. No sooner did she lift the receiver than she lost her place on the word processor. Just as she began picking up the thread of where she had left off in her typing, the phone would ring again, or two phones would ring in quick succession, and she was back where she had started, except now there was a rising sense of panic adding to her fluster, a realization that something was not quite right, that she was floundering at tasks she had taken for granted and which had been until recently second nature to her. She tried staying late to play catch-up. Her boss appreciated her going the extra yard, but her family didn't. The kids wanted to know where Mom was at dinnertime. And her husband, out of concern, was asking why she was so tired, preoccupied, and seemingly cut off from the family. Weekends were given over to sleep, a futile attempt at recharging the flagging cognitive batteries. And so it had gone for a year, Felicity's life slowly slipping out of kilter, the nourishing activities of family life, social pursuits, and gentle, leisurely walks sacrificed in an attempt to salvage her career. Still she refused to look reality in the face and admit the job was drifting away from her. The stakes were simply too high financially. Disability came with a one-third drop in earnings. Too tight a margin here. And then one day she is called in by a boss who she likes and who undoubtedly likes and respects her too, which is why he is looking so uncomfortable when he hands her a performance rating with those embarrassing adjectives that anger her even though she knows they are true.

I went through Felicity's cognitive results with her, test by test. I was sorry her husband was not with her to lend support, but he, too, is under pressure at work and could not take the afternoon off. It came as little comfort to her to know that memory and executive functioning were intact when processing speed was not. One essential cognitive domain was faulty. That is all it took to derail the whole process. Looking to the future, it is clear that accommodations at work are not an option. The company is not big enough to soak up the loss in time and productivity that this would entail. Longevity of service is appreciated, and there will be heartfelt and emotional farewells with no false sentiments hiding behind an oversized thank-you card, an expensive bottle of perfume, and a gorgeous floral arrangement a world away from the plastic replica that in truth always niggled at her. The tears that she sheds in my office will be shed again when she cleans out her desk and hugs those people she has been closest to at work. There will be promises to stay in touch, and to begin with they will be kept, albeit with increasingly long intervals between them as life gets in the way, until these too will falter, just as Felicity's processing speed did. One day, it will dawn on her that she has not seen her colleagues in ages, but this time she will not pick up the phone because she is always the one doing the phoning. That awareness is just too painful. Better to let the connections go.

Felicity is 39 years of age. All of her friends work. Her children are at school. Her husband is putting in long hours on a construction site. She sips her morning coffee alone in a silent house and wonders, What now? How did my life come to this? And with time on her hands, oodles of time, her mind drifts back to the day she was diagnosed with multiple sclerosis. Could she have foreseen where the disease would take her? She had always feared the wheelchair. That was her worse-case scenario. That is where her aunt, her mother's sister, had ended up. Well, 15 years on, it looked like she had cheated the wheels only to be floored by something she never could have envisaged. Slowed processing speed. Even her neurologist hadn't heard of it back then.

Let us now step out of the enforced quiet of the neuropsychologist's office with the "hush" sign hanging on the doorknob, asking passersby to be silent please because testing is in progress, and return to the real world. This move from quiet to unquiet is a major transition from a cognitive perspective. The divide is starkly revealed if we look at the life of Laura,

29 years of age with nine-year history of MS, who has been referred to my clinic by her neurologist because of struggles at work. Her position is, at first glance, a relatively simple one. She runs a checkout till in a large supermarket. She has done so for years. By all accounts, a routine job, keeping the conveyer belt moving and the cash register ringing.

Laura's social and medical histories explain her work career and why she is so determined to keep her job. Childhood was not a happy time for her. One of seven children, she was the middle child lost in the family shuffle. Dad was a drinker and a fierce disciplinarian who resorted to the strap; Mom was perpetually tired, anxious, and bullied. Money was always short, and the only topic the two seemed to agree upon was that the kids needed to get out and work as early as possible because that would take them off the books. Laura quit school at 16 years of age, against the advice of her teachers, one of whom tried telling her that she was a smart student with university potential. She never believed it. How could she when her father, smelling of rye, would tell her how stupid she was, reinforcing the message by whipping it into her with his belt? When she left school, Laura left the family home too, moving into a one-bedroom apartment with an older sister. To make ends meet, she put on a short, tight skirt and began serving in a raucous sports bar where the drink trumped the food and her job was to keep it that way.

The first symptoms of MS appeared when Laura was 20 years old: an altered sense of sensation from the waist down and some leg weakness. It made it difficult for her to maneuver between the tables in the bar, where space was tight, but she plowed on because she needed the money, and what alternatives were there with such a basic education? When her first relapse occurred two years later, the sensory symptoms worsened—it felt as though someone had tied a thick cord around her midriff and was pulling it tighter and tighter. The leg weakness deteriorated too, and she started to drag her legs. A few of the more boisterous and insensitive customers, noticing her labored gait, made fun of her. What hurt more than anything was when one man, and she remembers him well because of his heavy tattoos, teased her for being drunk and suggested she come with him to his Thursday rehab meetings where, he sniggered, you would always be guaranteed a good stiff drink. The boor smelled bad, just like her Dad—a mixture of cheap booze and stale sweat.

With work becoming increasingly difficult, Laura began looking around despondently for alternatives. A new megastore had just opened in the neighborhood and the supermarket side was hiring. She applied for a cashier position because it offered her the chance to sit all day. No matter that the pay was not quite as good as bar work. To be allowed to sit and work! What a relief. And, as a bonus, there were no more gibes, groping hands, or smutty invitations. Gone, too, was the stink of the alehouse, which seemed to work its way into her pores, defying a vigorous shower and scented shampoo. To be sure, the cashier work was not too exciting. If she really wanted to be honest with herself, it was actually boring, but she was allowed to sit on the job. That was the clincher. To sit and get paid while doing so. Oh yes, and no night work! She thanked her good fortune for landing the position. It was keeping her one step ahead of her disease.

Five years into her job, the company introduced a number of changes to enhance the customer's shopping experience, make the line-ups shorter, speed up the process, and lessen the time consumers spent in the store without reducing what they purchased. The consultants hired to revamp the "consumer experience" calculated the company could squeeze in up to 20% more shoppers during an 8 a.m. to 10 p.m. day, seven days a week, Christmas excluded. Simple math really, an algorithm that delighted the boardroom. The cashiers were integral to this. They would be required to take over pricing the fruit and vegetables that had up until then been priced by another employee who ran the booth with weights and scales in the midst of the produce section. Newer technology made the change possible. Laura was given a large computer screen with little icons for each food. When the customer dropped six peaches in front of her, she would look for the peach icon, tap it, and enter the number of peaches, and the amount would automatically be tallied before she moved on to the 3 potatoes, 12 bananas, and so on. It was corporate genius. Why have the produce weighed and priced in one place only to have the checkout person duplicate part of the process by zapping the barcode before the item was passed to the packer?

Cut out a step, trim redundancy, streamline the staff, reduce the wage bill, and as a bonus, speed up the works so that more was sold in less time. There was no matching increase in pay for the checkout staff. When one of them queried why, she was firmly reminded that no one was forcing her to stay. There was a long line of enthusiastic replacements just champing at the bit, didn't she know?

This change in how goods were priced seemed simple enough to Laura, but the funny thing was she had trouble with it. She couldn't quite keep up at times. Until then, her job had entailed moving the goods along the conveyer belt, finding and scanning all the barcodes, choosing debit over credit or vice versa, swiping a dizzying array of special points cards, bantering with the friendlier customers, smiling at their kiddies (even the obnoxious ones), calling her supervisor to come over when a barcode didn't show up or spat out nonsense figures, answering queries about where to find detergent or ice cream or laxatives, keeping the surfaces clean after a spillage (the processed fruit juices were the worst I learned because everything turned super-sticky if not wiped down properly), and all the while remaining friendly, helpful, and considerate, even when a customer who should have been at home in bed sucking on a eucalyptus lozenge sneezed all over her and coughed in her face. All of this had been fine and dandy, another day's work, another shift toward a modest paycheck, and all done thankfully while sitting down. But now, after only a single session of training, Laura was being asked to push a smorgasbord of icons, sometimes 30 or more if it was a big shop, and count the produce, which was not too bad with sizable oranges and grapefruit but far more challenging with little radishes and fresh figs. Her pace slackened. The conveyer belt slowed. The lines at her station grew longer. Customers began changing to lanes alongside hers. She heard them passing along advice to fellow shoppers lining up, clearly within earshot and oblivious to her presence: "Try another till. This one is really slow." After she botched one checkout, an irate customer called her a "retard" and asked to speak to the manager.

Looking back, Laura could see that the icons had been the tipping point. Just one more task, a time-dependent task in an attention span that was at capacity. How was she to know this? "How could a task so simple cause me so many problems?" she asked. The results of her neuropsychological testing gave her the answer, and it was bittersweet. Laura was surprised, stunned really, to learn that she had a pre-MS intelligence well above average. Prior to the onset of her MS, she had been, and indeed still was, a very intelligent person. MS had not dulled this. But MS had slowed her processing speed. Her results on the Symbol Digit Modalities Test (SDMT) were on the cusp of impaired. She could not complete the three-second Paced Auditory Serial Addition Test (PASAT-3), abandoning the task half way through when she simply could not keep up with the flow of digits. However, in a person of high intellect, low normal represented a major falloff in performance. The same could be said for many of her other cognitive indices. Verbal memory average, nonverbal memory low average, executive function low average. All within the normal spectrum but well below where she had once functioned. The challenging part, from an interpretive perspective, was to fathom why she could no longer function at work. After all, as she was quick to point out, her job was not an intellectually challenging one.

This case history illustrates a couple of interesting aspects of cognitive functioning in people with MS. The first point is directly linked to Laura's pre-MS intellectual abilities. As you will recall from the preceding chapter, this can be ascertained from a reading test, such as the Wechsler Test of Adult Reading. People with a high IQ—that is, those whose scores are above the general population mean, and in particular those with scores that are one standard deviation or more above the mean—have an inbuilt protective barrier to cognitive impairment. These are individuals with high *cognitive reserve*. A robust cognitive reserve does not confer immunity against cognitive decline, but it can soften the blow. Here it is important to remember that determination of impairment is a statistical construct. People with MS who are tested neuropsychologically have their scores compared to a normative data set obtained from healthy individuals matched according to sex, age, and years of education, three demographic variables that can influence cognition. Impairment thresholds can be set at different levels, but one that is frequently used is a decline of 1.5 standard deviations below the normative mean. Care must also be taken when interpreting results from individuals from disparate cultures and those whose ages fall above the typical upper limit of 60 (or 65) years taken as a standard point of reference for adult MS cognitive studies.

With this in mind, let us return to the SDMT. Here the normative mean for a healthy group of Canadian volunteers tested in my lab is 58.0 with a standard deviation of 10.8. A standard deviation of 1.5 equals 16.2 and, therefore, establishes the threshold for impairment at 41.8. Any individual whose score falls below this is considered impaired. This formula holds up well for the majority of people; that is, those with an average IQ. But what of that smaller group with a strong cognitive reserve? Given that they are starting at a higher baseline to begin with, a 1.5 standard deviation decline will not be enough to drop their scores below the threshold indicative of impairment. As such, they are classified intact, notwithstanding this decline. Laura, with her high pre-MS IQ, fell in this group.

Cognitive reserve is the product of intellectual enrichment and maximal lifetime brain growth (MLBG). The latter is estimated from head size or intracranial volume adjusted for sex. The protective effect of MLBG, synonymous with brain reserve, is based on the premise that people with larger MLBG can lose more brain volume (i.e., atrophy) before reaching the threshold at which cognitive deficits become apparent. In a series of elegant studies, James Sumowski and colleagues have shown how cognitive reserve can mitigate the effects of cerebral atrophy on cognitive performance.[1] The markers of intellectual enrichment are educational attainment and/or vocabulary. The environment in which one grows up is therefore a crucial formative influence. An enriched education boosts cognitive reserve and so does the pursuit of leisure activities.[2] "All work and no play makes Jack a dull boy. But all play and no work makes him something worse," declaimed Samuel Smiles, the Scottish author of *Self Help*, considered the bible of mid-Victorian liberalism. Looking beyond Smiles's moral opprobrium, contemporary neuroscience would agree. People with MS who are artists and musicians, however, may be disappointed to learn that, among an array of intellectually enriching activities, reading and writing were found to be more protective of memory.[3]

A five-year longitudinal study has confirmed the benefits of high cognitive reserve on SDMT performance.[4] One can therefore plausibly argue that in Laura's case, her high cognitive reserve was a key factor that allowed her to keep working until now. But, as we have also seen with Laura, there can still be real-world challenges even when a good cognitive reserve prevents an SDMT result from slipping below the threshold demarcating failure. Allied to her decline is another limiting factor, one that brings into focus one of the limitations of traditional neuropsychological testing—the ecological validity of the results. On the one hand, we have the tumult of the supermarket, on the other, the zen-like serenity of the tester's office. Polar opposites. Transplant the checkout counter with its new 18-inch monitor jam-packed—to use a good supermarket metaphor—with icons to the psychometrician's whisper-quiet office, conveniently situated out of the way off a corridor that sees little traffic, and it is likely that Laura would keep the counter scooting along briskly and her customers happy. However, the distractions of her regular working environment are considerable, and I have not even touched upon the Muzak that blares forth relentlessly, a medley of forced cheerfulness cranked out at decibels that can make you wince. For five years she had been able to function well in an environment overflowing with distractions, albeit at the limits of her capabilities. The icons had indeed been the tipping point, one more draw on her limited attention, which unbeknownst to her was already at capacity. Factor in the necessity for speed, and her neural networks, already challenged, could respond no faster even in the context of her high cognitive reserve.

The work travails of Laura illustrate the considerable challenges posed by distraction to a person whose cognitive abilities are already compromised. It is a situation that I encounter frequently in my MS clinic: the disconnect between cognitive results within the normal range and a work performance that fails to match this. With this observation, so often repeated, as a starting point, my research team set about trying to create a more "real world" environment during the testing process.[5] To do this, we returned to our computerized analog of the SDMT (described in Chapter 2; see figure 2.4) and embedded real-world distracters within it as follows: In line 2, a telephone rang; in line 5, a car horn went off; in line 7, a telephone rang again. Distracters were presented through an external speaker system attached to the computer at a standard level of 100 decibels. Each distracter lasted for eight seconds. Failure on the computerized SDMT analog was defined as a response time greater than a 1.5 standard deviation above the normative mean derived from healthy volunteers. Given that the sounds were computer controlled, they could be standardized. Thus, every participant heard the telephone and car horn for exactly the same duration and at the same volume. The aim in modifying the SDMT analog in this fashion was to replace the quiet of the testers office with a noisier environment geared toward distracting the person taking the test. We then administered the two versions of the SDMT analog to 99 people with MS and 55 healthy subjects. All participants also completed the traditional paper version the SDMT with responses recorded orally.

The results, which are displayed in figure 3.1, reveal the degree to which auditory distracters, when applied to a visual task, can slow performance, even in healthy control subjects. The slowing, however, is noticeably more marked in the people with MS. An incidental finding present in both the MS and healthy subjects is that performance on the

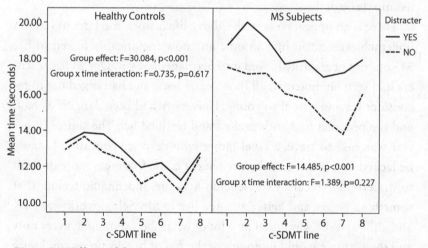

Figure 3.1. Effects of distraction on performance using a computerized Symbol Digit Modalities Test analog

computerized SDMT analog, even in the presence of distracters, speeds up over the course of the eight trials, a function of practice effects.

These distracter data become even more informative when we focus on those people with MS who have high cognitive reserve. When this group was given the traditional paper version of the SDMT, their failure rate was 30%. This jumped to 48% with the distracter SDMT analog, the 18% increase proving statistically significant. Most tellingly, 23% of individuals with high cognitive reserve who were cognitively intact on an array of additional cognitive measures, including the traditional SDMT, failed the distracter version. There are therefore certain individuals with MS with a high pre-MS IQ whose performances shift from normal on traditional tests done in a quiet environment to abnormal in the presence of these noisy distracters. One such person was Laura. She had more than enough innate intellectual ability to run her checkout counter. She was painfully aware of her colleagues at the other 20 tills having no problems managing the task, even with the icons added. After five years in the position, she was also cognizant, although hesitant to say to so, of being just as smart as the other women in the red-and-white maple-leaf aprons that sported the company's patriotic logo. What flummoxed her was an inability to retain focus and attention amidst a babble of voices, the clatter of trolleys, and that relentless wave of chipper, mindless music piped fortissimo through the store.

There is an upbeat coda to the above life history. It relates to Laura's underachievement in life, an outcome now inextricably linked to her MS but not necessarily locked into permanence by it. One of her teachers had seen her potential all those years back and had urged her to reconsider leaving school so young. University had been dangled as bait, and the prospect had both excited and terrified her. The source of her fear was easy to trace, a cruel father who despised education because he lacked any. But where the excitement came from was more difficult to discern. She recalls experiencing a vague, indefinable feeling that something bigger and better awaited her in life. Schoolwork was easy and although she was bored by a lot of what she was taught, every now and then a topic would jump out of the fog of her disinterest and seize her attention. History did that, particularly those periods in which her country found itself at war. The battles of 1812, the two world wars, Korea—she plunged into these topics with relish, trying to escape the battlefield of home-life with its slaps, punches, and drunken curses by immersing herself in another, less dangerous conflict, separated from harm by time, geography, and the pages of a book. She recalls an essay she wrote on the Canadians at Vimy Ridge. She spent all her afternoons in the library researching the topic. What a haven the place was, she recalls, and how difficult it had been to go home when evening fell and the librarians shooed her away from the racks. Her essay created something of a sensation. It won first prize in a school competition commemorating the First World War. Open to all high schoolchildren in her region, she remembers. Laura's teacher had her read her essay to the class and invited the principal down to hear it. Laura recollects the silence that greeted her final words and the odd look on the faces of her peers as they stared at her, not knowing what to make of what they had just heard. She can still feel the heat of embarrassment intermingled with pride when her principal began clapping and signaled the students to follow. It was then that her teacher made a final pitch to keep her in class. It amounted to a plea. But the cause was lost. Fear easily trumped nascent ambition. It was never really a contest. She was two months shy of her 16th birthday. MS was lying in wait, but how was she to know that?

I observe her closely as she reminisces. Twenty-nine years old, looks more like 40, petite, worry lines etched into a furrowed brow, tight lips a little dry from the side effects of her medication, no makeup, hair a tad greasy and pulled back tight into a short pony tail, faded denims and a clean, washed out khaki shirt hanging loose, a wedding band on her ring finger (it had been her grandma's, the only person in the family strong enough to stand up to Laura's father), scuffed sneakers, and a faux leather bag marked by heavy use. Money is tight and it shows. But so too does something else, a fighting spirit, a refusal to go under, a lovely smile that momentarily blots out the weariness and hurt and opens a window to an inner vibrancy of which she is unaware. She carries the scars of her childhood, corrosive to self-esteem and a barrier to personal insight.

Quitting school and leaving home did not put an end to the abuse. She swapped Dad for an assortment of men who treated her no differently. When her MS really started to show and her limp could no longer be camouflaged, her last boyfriend walked out on her, but not before getting hold of her bank card and cleaning out her checking account. She dug herself out of that one too, but now she is facing the biggest test of all, she tells me. She cannot keep her job at the supermarket. There are no accommodations to be had on the checkout counters. The conveyer belts run at one speed only. Fast.

"I have made bad choices," she confesses. "Chose the wrong men, left school too early, and now the MS is taking away my legs. What now? Where do I go from here?"

My answer floors her. Why not turn the clock back and think of college? She looks at me incredulously. When she does find her voice, there is a note of reproach in it. "This is unfair, Doc," she admonishes and begins listing all the perceived barriers to my suggestion. I wait for her to finish and then reply countering each of her arguments. A disability allowance will give her enough to live on. Her housing is already subsidized. Obtaining a high school diploma through adult education classes is free. She would need no more than a year to complete this. Universities offer part-time courses with accommodations to students with disabilities, and there are loans that the government offers prorated according to the student's financial needs. I remind her, "MS has not taken away your intelligence. It has slowed your processing speed, but you are still the same smart woman you once were when your principal praised you."

It took three further therapy sessions to break through the skepticism, but in the end, doubt gave way to enthusiasm. And I noticed that as Laura's misgivings faded, a subtle change became discernible in her mental state. The word that best describes it is lightness. The weight of the past lifted a little. Her smile was less forced, her face not so taught, her hair freshly washed and hanging loose. Money was still an issue, and living on the edge would never be conducive to a carefree demeanor, but to do something that you believed in, that stimulated you intellectually, with a goal on the horizon, was liberating. With accommodations in place, Laura raced through her catch-up high school year and enrolled part time in a Bachelor of Arts program at her local university, majoring in history. She understood that a three-year degree would take double the time, and no one knew what would come after that with a job and, more importantly, her health. But the uncertainties never fazed her. She had lived with them her whole life. MS was only one of them.

The MS-distraction literature is small in contrast to an extensive general neuropsychological one. And if we look beyond the purview of neuropsychology and behavioral medicine, we see that the subject has also excited the attention of the great novelists and poets.[6] In 1975, Nobel laureate Saul Bellow gave an address to the University of Chicago Board of Trustees. He chose as his subject "distraction," taking his cue from William Wordsworth's poem, "The World Is Too Much with Us," published in 1807. Life in England at the beginning of the nineteenth century was being rapidly transformed by the industrial revolution, and Wordsworth lamented what he saw as society in thrall to materialism, its citizens increasingly blind to the beauty of nature. "Getting and spending we lay waste our powers," he ruefully decried. Bellow took up Wordsworth's theme, noting that as the United States entered the last quarter of the twentieth century, "we have now a class of people who cannot bear that the world should not be more with them." While Bellow was primarily concerned with the place of the artist in the modern world, in his critique of contemporary society—"we are in a state of radical distraction"—and his skepticism that technology could "liberate us from the tyranny of noise and distraction," we also see the challenges facing the everyman.

These challenges come into even starker relief for the person with MS, as the data show. Moreover, the deleterious effects of distracters on processing speed in people with MS do not end here. They are magnified by another common condition that disproportionately affects people with the disease relative to the general population: depression. In a subsequent study of 102 people with MS, 30.6% of the sample who were not depressed failed the computerized SDMT analog without distracters, the figure rising to 50% in depressed participants and 73.3% in the presence of depression plus distracters.[7] This result takes on greater salience in the context of data showing that approximately one in two people with MS will develop a major depressive disorder over the course of their lives.[8] Daytime sleepiness as a consequence of insomnia, likewise common in people with MS, is associated with similar findings.[9] In light of these studies, it should come as no surprise to learn that Stefan van der Stigchel, professor of experimental psychology at Utrecht University, has concluded that we like to stare at a blank wall when we're thinking.[10]

Before leaving the topic of cognition and distracters, I would like to share the findings of one more study from my lab in which we approached the problem from a different angle.[11] The study involved the well-known gorilla-in-the-room experiment.[12] This celebrated cognitive teaser contains a short movie clip in which the viewer sees two groups of people wearing white or black T-shirts moving around and passing a ball within their respective groups. The viewer is asked to count the number of times the white team passes the ball. Unbeknownst to the viewer, a person wearing a gorilla suit enters the frame half way through the task, beats his chest and lingers briefly before moving out of view. Numerous studies have shown that healthy, well-educated people more often than not fail to see the gorilla, a normal phenomenon called inattention blindness. When people with MS and a healthy control group were administered a detailed cognitive battery including the gorilla paradigm, the people with MS were statistically more likely to see the gorilla. At first reading this might seem like a positive result for the MS group, but a closer look at some of the other cognitive data reveals a more worrying picture. Seeing the gorilla was associated with greater impairment on the Stroop Test, a classic distracter paradigm that also captures processing speed and executive functioning. Furthermore, the people with MS who struggled with the Stroop but who saw the gorilla also fared poorly when it came to accurately counting the number of ball passes made by the team wearing white. In short, the greater likelihood of seeing the gorilla was poor compensation for a cognitive profile characterized by heightened distractibility and impaired information processing speed.

The studies cited above indicate the challenges posed by distraction to people with MS. Healthy people are not immune to these challenges of course, but they will not be so profoundly affected by them. Most importantly, the disruptive effects of distraction to people with MS (and to those with acquired brain injuries in general) help explain, in part, why individuals who perform within normal limits on office-based neuro-psychological testing often fail to match that performance at work or in their homes.

The great poets and novelists do more than move us with words. Their keen insights into the human condition also coalesce with the work of empiricists. It would, however, be remiss not to counterbalance the concerns of Wordsworth and Bellow with the upside to our species' bumpy journey through time. Amidst the tumult of escalating distractions are to be found quantum advances that allow us to use the very devices of our distractibility—computers, tablets, and smart phones—to capture hitherto unimaginable real-time, real-world data and to develop tools for home-based detection and, most importantly, remediation of the cognitive deficits that cast such a long shadow. It is too soon to say whether these benefits will win out in the end. What is more certain, if literary history is our guide, is that distractions are not only here to say but will almost surely increase.

As mentioned previously, another advantage of the SDMT is that the test, or variations of it, can be readily administered via computer. To varying degrees, these computerized adaptations minimize the role of the tester, and in some instances dispense with the tester entirely. There are benefits that come with the latter approach. These include a completely standardized presentation that does not vary from person to person, fully automated scoring, and the potential to make the test far more widely available (e.g., by introducing it into medical offices and clinics where historically there has never, with a few exceptions, been a trained tester to administer neuropsychological tests). Doing away with a tester also saves money. Finally, by collecting sufficient normative data with the test, one can establish a threshold to define impairment. That cut-off number can then be built into the scoring algorithm so that the computer can instantly determine who has passed or failed the test.

These advantages are potentially offset by one major concern—the ability of a person who may be cognitively compromised to accurately and reliably test their own cognition. With this challenge in mind, a number of researchers have come up with their own fully automated variations on an SDMT theme. A team at the Cleveland clinic[13] developed an iPad-administered test of processing speed analogous to the cardinal feature of the SDMT; that is, matching numbers and symbols as quickly and accurately as possible in a set time period. The iPad Processing Speed Test (PST) was then administered to a group of people with MS who had also completed the paper and pencil SDMT and undergone a brain MRI. The results were impressive. The PST was found to have excellent test-retest reliability, correlated significantly with the traditional SDMT, was slighter better than the traditional SDMT in differentiating people with MS from healthy participants, and correlated strongly with lesion burden on MRI. Most importantly, the results obtained were the same irrespective of the presence of a tester in the room during the assessment.

One limitation to the test is the reliance on relatively intact neurological function to compete the test. People with MS had to have intact sensation, strength, and coordination in their hand to touch the matching symbol-number pairs on the iPad. It was for this reason that the test was compared to the pencil and paper version of the SDMT rather than the more widely used oral version. In addition, given the possibility of some individuals with MS having motor, sensory, and coordination deficits, the duration of time to complete the PST test was extended from 90 seconds, which is the conventional SDMT duration, to 120 seconds. The authors concluded that the iPad-administered PST was a practical tool for routinely screening processing speed deficits in people with MS.

An alternative approach to an iPad platform is one that relies on voice recognition. Working with colleagues in the Engineering Department at the University of Toronto, my research team took the computerized SDMT and modified the administration to allow for voice recognition, thereby dispensing with the tester entirely.[14] I have described the core features of the computerized SDMT previously when discussing the role of incidental memory in the SDMT and again when I gave details of the distracter experiments. When it came to adding the voice recognition component, no distracters were included and the symbol-digit code was kept fixed as in the traditional version of the test.

The voice recognition SDMT analog runs within Google's Chrome browser, on a Windows or MacOS-based computer that must be equipped with a reasonable quality microphone and audio speakers. The program consists of a user interface paired with a speech recognition module that accepts audio input to the test. The speech recognition module makes use of Google's online speech recognition service. The test works as follows: the participant sits in front of the computer screen and clicks the mouse to start. The computer begins by asking the person for basic demographic information (age, sex, total years of education) before going on to administer an eye test to make sure the individual has adequate (20/70) vision. Should the person fail the eye test, the program terminates. If the person passes, the computer proceeds to administer the voice recognition SDMT analog. In the instruction phase, the individual is required to successfully complete a practice trial before starting the test. This provides a measure of the person's oral-motor ability. With this preparatory stage completed, the person is then administered the full test. A video of the test can be viewed at vr-pst.com. The computer records the time per line completed, the total time for all eight lines completed, the mean time for the eight trials and the total number of errors made.

The percentages of MS participants impaired on the voice recognition SDMT analog and the traditional oral SDMT were 34% and 32%, respectively. Excellent convergent validity was found between the two tests, both in people with MS and healthy participants (figure 3.2). Interestingly, 70% of people with MS and healthy participants preferred being tested by a computer than a person, but the study was not designed to explore reasons for this. The voice recognition version had a similar sensitivity and specificity to the traditional oral SDMT in predicting overall cognitive impairment on the Brief International Cognitive Assessment in MS (BICAMS). And while the BICAMS refers here to tests that were administered by a tester, there is now preliminary evidence that the entire battery is also effective as a screening tool when

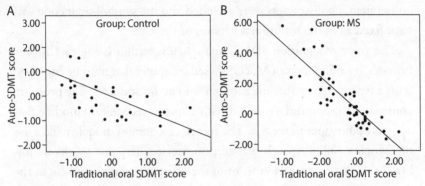

Figure 3.2. Comparison of performance on the fully automated SDMT analog versus the traditional oral SDMT in healthy controls (*A*) and people with MS (*B*)

given digitally and unsupervised.[15] With rapid technological advances giving impetus to the field, a burgeoning literature reveals an array of computerized tests and cognitive batteries that have entered, or are about to enter, clinical practice.[16]

When it comes to the treatment of impaired processing speed, results from pharmacologic interventions using stimulant medications, such as L-amphetamine, methylphenidate, and modafinil, are mixed and at times contradictory. In a literature bedeviled by methodological short-comings, most notably a paucity of studies with cognitive variables as a primary outcome measure, the yield to date from disease-modifying therapies (DMTs) has been modest, at best. A meta-analysis of 41 studies involving 7,131 people with relapsing-remitting MS reported a small to moderate positive effect on cognition, mostly within the domain of processing speed.[17] No difference in cognitive benefits were present between platform (mainly interferon-β and glatiramer acetate) and escalation (natalizumab and fingolimod) therapies. At first glance, this finding can be misleading. The processing speed finding is not indicative of DMTs having a selective, beneficial effect on this aspect of cognition. Rather, it reflects the emergence of the SDMT as a central cognitive measure in this population with clinical trials often including it as the lone cognitive test, tacked on as a secondary or tertiary outcome measure in a study where the primary points of interest are markers of neurological function such as the Expanded Disability Status Scale (EDSS) or clinical relapse and MRI indices of disease activity. More impressive in this regard is a recent double-blind, placebo-controlled, phase-3 trial of siponimod in people with secondary progressive MS. The beneficial effects of DMT treatment on the SDMT, but not the PASAT and a test of visual memory, were found after 12 months of therapy.[18]

Equivocal conclusions characterize the dalfampridine data with positive effects on the SDMT from one class I trial offset by negative results from class II and III trials (see Chen et al., 2020, for a comprehensive review of the pharmacologic literature in general).[19] Interestingly, given its repurposed use, potentially more promising cognitive results have emerged from a 24-month trial of simvastatin, once more in people with secondary progressive MS.[20]

Which brings us back to computers. Not only do they aid in neuropsychological assessments, they may be opening the way to effective treatment options when processing speed falters. A number of studies have shown benefits for an array of computerized programs.[21-24] Of particular interest is that improvements have been reported for people with more advanced disease—namely, secondary progressive[25]—and for those who completed the program at home.[26] Researchers have also creatively harnessed the potential of computers and developed video games that can improve SDMT performance.[27,28] All of these computerized interventions are relatively brief, administered over four to eight weeks depending on the particular program. As such, benefits tend to accrue quickly.

While approaches such as these are potentially promising, a number of big, unanswered questions remain. First and foremost is to what degree do these changes elicited in a research setting translate into real-world benefits? This is of crucial importance and the answer is not yet known. There are hints that improvements may boost day-to-day functioning[22] but not quality of life.[26] With data being paltry, a lot more research is needed with a different set of outcomes, ones that tap into the practical challenges that people with MS confront in their daily lives. Some encouraging, preliminary work with virtual reality may bridge this divide.[29] A second question is do the benefits endure? While preliminary data suggest improvements may still be present six months after completing an intervention based on a personalized App,[21] the majority of studies do not contain such post-treatment follow-up data. And allied to this point are the questions of whether it is necessary for people with MS to continue the intervention to maintain benefits and, if so, for how long?

These important questions are not unique to processing speed interventions. As we will see in the following chapters, they apply equally to programs that address memory and executive function. However, these are relatively early days in an approach that potentially holds much promise. To date, Felicity and Roger have not had the trajectory of their lives shift with time-limited interventions like these. There has been no longed-for return to the kind of work they loved and were good at. Susan, on the other hand, was able to go to work as a pharmacist, albeit in a quieter, slow-paced position far removed from her dream of being in the vortex of a busy general hospital. As pointed out, however, outcomes like these must be viewed in the context of an inevitable response heterogeneity, for people with MS will respond differently, including some not at all, to these types of interventions.[30] But there is no doubt that computers and technology are transforming what had been a moribund field. Not too long ago, two Cochrane Reviews concluded there was weak evidence supporting cognitive rehabilitation for people with MS.[31,32] Now, opinions are shifting, as a systematic review and meta-analysis of the computerized cognitive-training literature makes clear.[33] While it is premature to predict a new dawn, a cautious, realistic element of hope is stirring for people with MS. There is much work to be done, but how much better to embark on a challenging journey buoyed by promising preliminary data and energized by a newfound optimism.

FOUR

Learning and Memory

MEMORY IMPAIRMENT, TO varying degrees of severity, affects approximately 60% of people with multiple sclerosis.[1] This broad statement, however, requires clarification for there are many different types of memory and not all of them are involved equally. One major subdivision splits memory into declarative and procedural components. The former requires effort and is therefore conscious, whereas the latter is not and is thus considered automatic. We use procedural memory, for example, when we ride a bike or open a door. These actions are done without having to pre-think them. This instinctive motor memory is learned through priming, conditioning, practice, and repetition, and it is generally spared in people with MS. Declarative memory, on the other hand, is often impaired, but further clarification is required once again because this too encompasses different subtypes such as working memory, semantic memory, and episodic memory.

Semantic memory refers to memory for facts and is generally intact in people with MS. Examples here are general knowledge questions like "What is the capital of Canada?" or "Who is the president of the United States?" Working memory refers to a cognitive system that is responsible

for the short-term maintenance and manipulation of information necessary for the performance of tasks such as learning, comprehension, and
reasoning.[2] A useful computer analogy is to consider working memory
as that information which is held online. Approximately one-third of
people with MS will show deficits in their use and manipulation of this
fund of briefly stored and frequently updated information. An example
of a cognitive test that probes working memory is the Digit Span Test,
one of the components of the Wechsler Adult Intelligence Scale–Revised.[3]
There is a Digits Forward and Digits Backward part to the Digit Span
Test. In the first, a tester reads aloud a sequence of numbers paced at one
per second. The subject has to repeat the number sequence exactly as
given. When the subject repeats the span length correctly, and two
chances are allowed for each span length, the tester increases the span
length by one digit. The test continues until the subject fails both trials or
a nine-digit span length is correctly repeated. The procedure is the same
for Digits Backward, except the subject has to repeat exactly the digit
span in reverse order. The test continues until the subject fails a pair of
sequences or recalls eight reversed digits correctly. Digits Backward is
clearly the more difficult of the two tasks and a sensitive marker of
working memory.

A test of working memory that is widely used in MS research and
clinical practice is the Paced Auditory Serial Addition Test (PASAT),[4]
described in Chapter 2. If you remember, it is also a test of processing
speed. To recall, participants listen to a series of numbers presented to
them at a set speed. They are instructed to add each new digit to the
one that preceded. Part of the challenge lies in giving the tester the correct total, while at the same time remembering the last digit to add to
the next one. This ability to remember the last number taps into working memory.

Another frequently used test of working memory is the n-back.[5] In
this test, the individual is shown a sequence of letters on a computer
screen. For the 0-back task, which is essentially a control task, they are
asked to click a mouse or push a button on a button box as quickly as
they can, when a designated letter, in this case "x," appears (figure 4.1A).

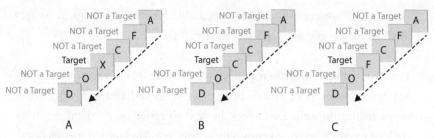

Figure 4.1. The n-back task: examples of 0-back (*A*), 1-back (*B*), and 2-back (*C*) tasks

In the 1-back task, the instruction is to push the button when a letter repeats itself (figure 4.1B). Remember that each letter disappears after it has been presented, so the individual is required to remember the preceding letters, which in the case of the 1-back, goes back at one letter. In the 2-back, the instruction is to push the button when a letter repeats itself, twice removed (figure 4.1C). There is a 3-back sequence as well, but in general MS researchers stop at the 2-back because the test is already quite challenging by this point. The n-back is ideally suited for presentation to a person while they are undergoing a functional MRI scan. The brain activations captured by the MRI illustrate the neural network that underpins working memory in healthy people, which has been well mapped,[6] and the degree to which this network might become disrupted in someone with a disease like multiple sclerosis. I will return to the brain imaging changes associated with memory impairment in people with MS later in this chapter.

The one type of memory that is most frequently affected in people with MS is episodic memory. This is best conceptualized as memory for specific events or situations. What did I eat for dinner last night? Who did I socialize with last week? What did my boss ask me to do this afternoon? When people with MS start forgetting things like this, it is not difficult to appreciate how much harder life can get. In the MS literature, the tests most frequently used to assess episodic memory are the California Verbal Learning Test,[7] which is part of the Minimal Assessment of Cognitive Function in MS (MACFIMS), and the Selective Reminding

Test,[8] which is part of the Brief Repeatable Neuropsychological Battery (BRNB) for people with MS (see Chapter 2).

The man sitting tensely in my office used to work as a director of a large Bay Street investment house. Brett is 41 years old and in his prime, he keeps telling himself. Last week he had to retire on medical grounds. He looks well. Everyone keeps telling him that. He has a vigorous handshake. He strides the long hospital corridors, easing past patients, visitors, and staff. He looks in a hurry, and for a time he was, as his career soared and he shot up the corporate ladder to his own office on the 64th floor of a gleaming skyscraper, where from a plush swivel chair he would take in the breathtaking view of the lake and islands below. He was widely acknowledged by his peers as a financial whiz, a prodigy who combined precocious ability with an uncanny sense of timing and foresight when it came to navigating the financial markets. Money was his commodity, large sums of money, and there are many people in this sprawling city and beyond who think of him fondly when they come to review their investment portfolios.

Five years back, Brett was diagnosed with MS. He never broke stride. A tough bit of news to get, but hey, the markets were tough too, and they could be tamed. He never ignored his disease, but in reality, once his initial weakness and numbness had resolved, it didn't trouble him. He recalls receiving his diagnosis in the midst of a bull market, the DOW surging, the Nasdaq at a record high, and all this heady excitement and stuffed corporate coffers sure took the sting out of what the neurologist had said. His one concession to the disease was a daily injection, a disease-modifying drug that came with no side effects other than a little bruising out of sight beneath the bespoke suit.

When the markets plunged, Brett's personal reputation soared—a paradox that was not lost on him—for he had unerringly positioned portfolios in a way that softened his investors' pain. As I got to know him a little better, I could see that he combined a keen intelligence with a canny ability to read people, which must surely have helped when it came to managing the livelihoods of clients with widely different appetites for risk. Along the way, he had looked after his own interests as well, building a way of life that would continue for his wife and two young boys even as he gave up his eagle's nest and confronted life far removed from the adrenaline-soaked world of the financial markets.

Outside of work, he played hard too. There was the golf club membership, the kind with a long wait list where you had to be put up to be considered, the cottage in the lake district, a speed boat moored alongside the dock, and the monthly single-malt club with a firm circle of friends who dated back to their time together at an all-male private school. A scripted life in so many ways but one. MS. While the fates had smiled kindly on him, blessing Brett with good looks, a strong cognitive reserve, and an outgoing, infectious temperament, there was no escaping his genes. An older cousin with MS used a wheelchair. An uncle with MS walked with a cane. A great-grandfather, diagnosis unclear, but presumed to be MS in hindsight, had not walked for the last half of his life. When Brett's number was called, he thought he had escaped the mobility aids, and he had this far. Where he had not dodged the bullet was with his episodic memory.

The onset of Brett's memory difficulties was subtle. Momentary forgetfulness was how he described it. He had had a first-rate personal assistant. She picked up his first big mistake, and he had teasingly thanked her by saying he owed her a large diamond and then some. When the next mistake was detected, she teased him back, asking if the diamond came with a broach. He laughed, a little uneasily this time, and had the florist deliver a beautiful arrangement instead. The third mistake was missed, and there was no humor this time, just an angry client who only six months back had been all smiles and bonhomie. Such was Brett's world. A decimal in the wrong place, a misplaced zero overlooked, and shock, surprise, rage, and sometimes worse, quickly followed.

Things started to unravel quickly after this. A call comes through from a long-standing client, now incandescent with rage. Why, he bellowed, had his instructions for a stock purchase not been followed? Brett cannot remember having had the discussion and at first pushes back against the charge of sloppiness. But late that evening, sifting through old emails, he finds the paper trail. His client finds it too, triggering a fresh fusillade. A week later, the experience is repeated with another client.

News travels fast in Brett's world. Large sums of money focus the mind, sharpen attention. Momentary forgetfulness in the financial world is not forgotten. It may be forgiven if the losses are recouped elsewhere, but that is not possible here. The markets are in the doldrums. A couple of the senior partners drop in for a chat, their expressions pained. His confidence shaken, Brett begins staying late at work, checking and double-checking the day's transactions. He has his PA take notes in meetings and type them up for him to go over at day's end. He takes to spending his evenings alone in his office, the entire floor now darkened, deserted, and still, the lights of a great metropolis twinkling below, the sounds filtering up off the street dwindling as the city empties. A scotch on the rocks in some convivial bar, the laughter of his boys before bedtime, a hug from his wife have given way to solitude and worry, a deep gut-wrenching worry that something is seriously amiss.

At times the disconnect between his recollection of the day's events and what his PA has transcribed is startling. Had he really told one client to sell? Another to buy? A third to sit tight? Well, he trusts his PA implicitly, and when he follows her script rather than his faltering memory, the angry telephone calls stop for a while. But the situation is not sustainable. He cannot rerun everything, constantly second guess himself, record and check every single item on a lengthy to-do list. There are situations where sticky notes fail as memory aids, where his PA cannot sit in on conversations, where he is forced to fly solo, and it is then, to continue with the aviation metaphor, that he crashes, and a crash in his world is not some minor peccadillo, coming as it does with all those damn zeros trailing after the dollar signs.

It takes 18 months before Brett comes see me. During this period, he tries very hard to right the ship of his failing cognition. Weekends at the cottage are sacrificed. Work is brought home and taken on vacations. A second PA is roped in as an early warning system, someone whose job it is to shadow his decisions and provide backup when needed. To begin with, this human buffer works well. Mistakes are caught early and corrected, and the investors are left smiling. But detecting errors is only one part of the problem. Intact episodic memory is necessary to drive other aspects of cognition, like decision making. The whole process of planning and deciding what to do, which in Brett's case involves an element of prediction as well, is underpinned by memory. Counteracting impaired memory is therefore much more than simply detecting errors. Errors might be the public face of a memory in trouble, but the subtler manifestations show up as actions, plans, and decisions that are not necessarily inaccurate but less innovative, creative, and insightful instead. Choices driven by a compromised memory may therefore turn out to be the lesser of two correct options. Decisions like these when repeated undermine client confidence. Relationships forged over a decade start to splinter. Here, the overlap with another aspect of cognition—executive functioning—becomes apparent and will be discussed in the next chapter. But for now, let us stay with episodic memory. A minor memory slip in the morning may prove inconsequential. So, too, another in the afternoon. But what if the two are linked? What if the two lapses coalesce, their summation proving greater than each individual part? And what if this cumulative forgetfulness generates a less than optimum decision about a particular share trade or stock option? The devil is in the details, is it not? Fudge the details, forget one or two of them, throw in a few million dollars, and you have the perfect storm.

Two years on from his first major mistake, Brett applies for disability based on his poor memory. It is an agonizing decision. Not only is he forced to concede that he can no longer function in the high-stakes environment of an investment firm, he also has to face the skepticism of some of his peers. After a break at his cottage, he returns trim and tanned, exuding good health, and sees their bemusement when he cites MS as the reason for his premature retirement. He hears the occasional snigger and is aware of rumors that he no longer has the right stuff. "Now you find out who your true friends are," he ruefully confides.

Poor episodic memory is the undoing of a high-flying investment analyst. It also lays low Mary, a stay-at-home mother with three young children. The history I obtain from her reveals she grew up in a happy middle-class family, a "traditional kind of family" is the way she describes it, in which Dad went to work each day at the Ford Motor Company assembly plant while Mom stayed home to raise the three kids. They were never rich, but her parents were prudent with money so that when Dad turned 65, he could take retirement, the mortgage already paid and the children on their way. It was a comfortable, uncomplicated path through life, a model Mary aspired to and thought she had achieved until MS intruded. She is in her early 30s, and life until recently had been a happy blur of getting her three kids up in the morning, organizing breakfast, seeing her husband off to the very same Ford production line, running a school car pool, shopping for groceries, keeping the house spotless, and grabbing a cup of coffee with a friend before starting the afternoon whirl of extracurricular activities, karate, piano lessons, ballet, and badminton. By the time hubby came home around six o'clock, the children were wrapping up their homework, dinner was in the oven, and a quiet evening lay in store. Mary ran a tight ship, just like her mother had, and she took pride in it. Everyone was happy. Life was good.

Then one morning Mary wakes up feeling dizzy. Her husband has to get the kids off to school because she gets an urgent appointment with her GP, who immediately refers her to the local ER. Before the day is out, a friend has to fetch the children from school and there is takeout for dinner because Mary is in bed and on the phone to a friend of hers who is a nurse, trying to make sense of whether she does or does not have MS. The way the diagnosis was broken was hurried and confusing, she recalls.

Things are a little topsy-turvy after that, but a course of steroids helps, and a month later Mary's dizziness is 90% better. A minor irritant, that's all. When her left arm goes weak a year later, the diagnosis of MS is confirmed, but steroids help again, and now the disease-modifying injections start every second day, which takes a little getting used to. Life is moving at such a quick tempo with three children, however, that the focus is soon off the needles and on to the after-school curriculum, which is busier than ever. Mary counts herself fortunate because, despite the diagnosis, she is feeling okay and seems to have escaped her worst fears. A little left-sided weakness, minimal dizziness—she can live with that. Routine is the order of business, the day mapped out like a military campaign, just like it always has been, the only change being coffee time is now replaced by a nap because fatigue cannot be ignored.

Two years pass, and then odd things start happening. Mary is at home having just woken from her snooze when the telephone rings. The call is from the orthodontist's office. She has missed an appointment with her youngest daughter. The news surprises her. She consults her diary and sees that it is true. All she can do is apologize and pay the fee. A month later, she receives a call from one of the school secretaries asking where she is and telling her not to worry because her kids will remain safely in the office until she gets there. She looks at her watch. It is midday. There must be some mistake. School ends at 2:30 p.m. Well, not today apparently. It's a half day, did she not remember? That night she has to break up an argument between her two youngest children. They are fighting over a tube of toothpaste. "Stop it, you each have your own," she admonishes them, only to find out they don't and have not for the past few weeks. "We kept telling you, Mom. Don't you remember?" "Nonsense," she replies, and goes in search of her husband. He will arbitrate here. Instead, she gets a hug, and he takes her into the den, closes the door and tells her gently that things are falling apart a little at home. He has been trying to help on the quiet by going to the convenience store to purchase items she has been missing at the supermarket. The toothpaste, however, escaped him too. She wants to know how long has this been going on for. His answer floors her. "About a year."

The ability to correctly appraise one's own memory is called metamemory, and metamemory is often impaired in people with MS. Mary's incredulity at being told by her husband of her difficulties is an example of this. Research has shown that people with MS who perceive their cognition as impaired are more likely to be depressed than to have objective evidence of cognitive deficits. While some individuals with the disease are aware of their cognitive failings, most do not have good insight into the presence of deficits or an awareness of the full extent of their deficits. Here, informants are usually better judges of cognition, providing the informant has had regular, close, and prolonged contact with the person with MS.

These observations were clearly demonstrated in an informative study undertaken by Ralph Benedict in Buffalo, New York. He designed and validated a self-report measure for cognitive dysfunction, the Multiple Sclerosis Neuropsychological Questionnaire, or MSNQ.[9] It is the only psychometric scale of its kind in the MS literature. There are two versions of the scale, one for the person with MS, the other for an informant. Each contains 15 simple questions and takes only a few minutes to complete. Benedict had a group of people with MS and their informants answer their respective set of 15 questions and then administered detailed neuropsychological testing to the people with MS. The results were unequivocal. Informant scores on the MSNQ correlated more robustly with the objective cognitive test results than the subjective responses of people with MS. Elevated MSNQ scores in those with MS, indicative of prominent cognitive complaints, correlated instead with depression.

The other side of the coin is true too. People with MS who report that their cognition is fine may not be accurate in their self-assessment, as the following care history shows. Doug is 39 years old and living back at home with his elderly parents after his wife left him a couple of years back. He has a mild degree of stiffness, which makes it a little more difficult to walk long distances. But walking, which is modestly challenging, is not the reason he has come to see me. Not only has he lost his wife but his work as a salesperson has ended too. He was fired because he was making too many mistakes. A couple of minutes into the interview and the reason for the company's punitive decision, which is now before a human rights arbiter, is soon obvious. He cannot tell me when he was diagnosed with MS. He has forgotten the names of his medications. He cannot remember how often to take them. He is not sure of when his work in sales ended. Each answer, heavy with uncertainty, is given arduously with a look of mild perplexity on his face, eyes darting to his father for confirmation or help. His level of memory impairment is obviously severe; the results of a neuropsychological assessment are merely confirmatory.

There is a deep poignancy to the interview. Doug is young. In the space of a couple of years he has lost his marriage, his job, his independence, and all his friends. His future was once bright. Now he needs his parents to look after him for he struggles with his banking, cannot earn a living, cannot even remember to return from the supermarket with the correct items purchased. He is an only child, and his parents had him late in life. His father, who is an invaluable informant, could pass for his grandfather. He, too, is not well—I can see the telltale signs of emphysema, the shortness of breath, heaving chest, and blueish tinge to the mouth. Doug's mother has her own health problems—diabetes has hobbled her, and that is why she is not at the appointment with them. They are devoted parents, their child a late-life blessing. And now this. The father looks at his son laboring away to remember such simple things, and you can see the pain in his expression, the deep concern on his face that reads like an open book. "What will become of my boy after I am gone?" he is wondering.

The usual case scenario of the child caring for an elderly, infirm parent has been upended here. Now it is the elderly parents who are the caregivers. They have become their son's memory as his recall falters and recollections fade. Such is his level of dysfunction they are leery of having him leave the house on his own. He recently went for a short walk, I am told. "Just around the block," he cheerfully reassured his parents before setting out. It was one of those glorious sunny late-September days, the heat and humidity of summer replaced by a delicious coolness that bathed the burnished gold and copper foliage. How could they not let him step outside to enjoy it all? Somewhere along the way, Doug took a left instead of a right turn and got lost. When the officer found him hours later, Doug was sitting on a park bench, eyes closed with a gentle smile on his face, caught in a warming shaft of afternoon sunlight. The officer had felt guilty disturbing him, until she remembered the distraught parents back home.

In the midst of this family tragedy, central to it all, sits Doug, in good spirits, oblivious to his cognitive losses. His metamemory is shot, and his awareness of his multiple failings is poor. You might argue that this is a blessing, for what good would it serve him to have full insight into the depth of his disability? However, Doug's anosognosia, or lack of insight, comes with a heightened vulnerability to a host of risks that range from personal safety issues, such as leaving the stove on or the bath taps running, to financial exploitation and manipulation. Doug is blithely unaware of all of this. His father is not. With Dad's health failing, the talk turns to establishing a trust fund to ensure a modest monthly income for his son. With an eye on the future, a search is also on for appropriate, supervised housing, a difficult task when the person to be housed is so young and the facilities designed to look after those with memory impairment are filled with a geriatric population struggling with Alzheimer's disease.

Laying down a new memory and then accessing it entails a sequence of tasks, encoding followed by consolidation and then retrieval. Each may be selectively impacted, and there is an ongoing debate in the MS neuropsychological literature as to which stage is most affected. For example, problems with memory are more prominent on tests of recall as opposed to recognition, suggesting the difficulty is mainly one of retrieval and not encoding.[10] In support of this, Rao et al.[11] administered a wide array of memory tests, which included, among others, Digit Span, Selective Reminding Test, Story Recall, and Free Verbal Recall, to 37 people with MS and 26 healthy people. Their results revealed that the memory impairment in people with MS arose from a diminished ability to access information already learned, whereas encoding and storage capacity were intact.

A dissenting view emerged five years later in a study by DeLuca et al.,[12] who showed that people with MS required significantly more trials to learn a new task than healthy individuals, but once learned, delayed retrieval between the two groups was similar. Twenty-five years later, the same lab returned to the topic and confirmed not only that encoding and early consolidation were affected in memory-impaired people with MS but also that it was linked with a decline in processing speed as measured on the Symbol Digit Modalities Test (SDMT).[13] The latter finding was not new.[14] Furthermore, the DeLuca group was not alone in asserting that the problem lay with encoding and consolidation, rather than retrieval. Other researchers had reached similar conclusions,[15,16] also noting an association with the degree of demyelination involving prefrontal fiber pathways seen on MRI.[17]

Multiple sclerosis is a multifocal disease. You will recall from Chapter 1 that a hallmark clinical characteristic of the disease, pivotal to the diagnosis, is that of damage to the central nervous system disseminated in space and time. In terms of memory, important *spaces* are the hippocampus and thalamus, both of which are deep gray matter structures. An appreciation of cortical and deep gray matter involvement in MS is relatively new. Neuropathology led the way[18,19] with subsequent in vivo confirmation coming from brain imaging.[20,21]

The thalamus is situated on both sides of the third ventricle. It relays the transmission of information between cortical and subcortical regions and, as such, plays a key role in sensory, motor, cognitive, and integrative functions.[22] Thalamic gray matter lesions,[23] subcortical gray matter demyelination,[24] and thalamic atrophy[25] have all been reported in MS.

A brief digression is helpful here, lest we forget history and by way of reintroducing the thalamus into a discussion on memory. In 1985, just before MRI became widely available clinically, researchers reported that brain atrophy as measured by CT scan was associated with impairments in memory and verbal intelligence.[26] Atrophy was measured in different ways, and the imaging parameter that was found to be most robustly linked to memory impairment was the width of the third ventricle. Furthermore, data showed that memory worsened with increasing atrophy of the third ventricle, as we can see in figure 4.2.

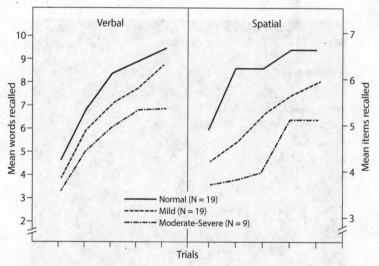

Figure 4.2. The relationship between degrees of third ventricle atrophy and verbal and nonverbal (spatial) memory impairment in people with progressive MS. See ref. 26 in chap. 4.

This imaging study is notable for two things. The first is the absence of any mention of the hippocampus in relation to the presence of memory impairment. This omission reflects the limitations of CT, which lacks the spatial resolution of MRI and is confined to scanning in the axial plane, thereby precluding good visualization of the medial temporal lobes which house the hippocampus. The second notable point is that it provided early evidence of the role played by the thalamus in cognition, for third ventricle width is a surrogate measure of thalamic volume: the smaller the thalamus (figure 4.3), the wider the ventricle.

This finding was replicated with MRI by Benedict et al.,[27] who confirmed the primacy of third ventricle width over other markers of brain atrophy (brain parenchymal fraction, bi-caudate ratio) and lesion volume as a predictor of numerous cognitive indices, including slower processing speed and verbal and visual memory impairment. In turn, this finding was extended by Houtchens et al.,[28] who obtained multiple neuroimaging metrics including lesion volume, brain parenchymal fraction, third ventricle width, and a direct measure of thalamic volume, and who concluded that the latter correlated most robustly with multiple aspects of cognition, including memory.

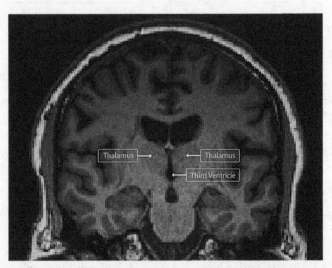

Figure 4.3. The relationship of the third ventricle to the thalamus

The hippocampus resembles a seahorse and is found within both temporal lobes. It is subdivided into sections—CA1, CA2/CA3, CA4, and so on—each of which is specialized in terms of function.[29] The hippocampus can be affected in many different ways in MS. Demyelinating lesions[30] and a reduction in neurons[31] are common. There are fewer neuronal synapses within demyelinated areas leading to reduced neuronal transmission.[32] In addition, atrophy may occur as a consequence of local damage from inflammatory and degenerative changes and as a secondary, indirect process via a reduction in hippocampal connections to other brain regions.[33]

There is evidence that certain regions of the hippocampus, such as CA1 and the subiculum, are particularly susceptible to damage in people with MS.[34,35] This in turn is more likely to be associated with deficits in learning and memory, both for verbal and nonverbal material.[36] Damage to regions CA2/3 and the dentate gyrus, on the other hand, is more closely linked to symptoms of depression[37] (see Chapter 8). These associations between regional hippocampal damage and behavioral change have been elucidated by numerous MRI studies which reinforce the central role of the hippocampus in networks of connected structures that underpin memory. For example, in an MRI and cognitive study of 32 people with MS and 16 healthy subjects, detailed structural (lesions, atrophy) and functional (activation during an episodic memory task) data were obtained from the hippocampus and thalamus.[38] The results showed that immediate recall on a visual-spatial task was significantly associated with hippocampal volume, whereas as delayed recall on the same task associated more closely with thalamic volume. Notably, functional activation of the thalamus during encoding was more predictive of memory impairment than the volumetric measurements.

The importance of hippocampal network connectivity to verbal and visuospatial memory was confirmed in a study of 71 people with MS and 50 healthy participants.[39] Intact structural connectivity between the hippocampus on the one hand and the thalamus, insula, and occipital cortex on the other also emerged as necessary for maintaining episodic memory. Allied to the structural integrity of neural networks is the concept of brain dynamics, which refers to the *strength* of communication between relevant network hubs or nodes. Evidence here suggests a laterality effect with lower dynamic functional connectivity of the left and right hippocampi associated with verbal and visuospatial memory deficits respectively.[40]

The relative importance of the hippocampus and thalamus and their connections to the neural networks underpinning memory will vary according to the type of memory assessed and the particular cognitive tests used, as the studies referenced here reveal. When damaged, the impairments that ensue will leave their mark on people with MS in many different ways: an inability to find or sustain work, frayed relationships, financial hardship, an inability to drive, and heightened safety concerns, among others. Should the deficits be severe, the ramifications can be devastating and come into stark relief when social factors have removed the safety net that could have softened the blow. The following case history illustrates this point.

What happens when you don't have parents, siblings, extended family, or friends to look out for you? When you are still young and have retained your boyish good looks and your body remains strong even as your memory progressively slips? When those two little letters, MS, seem at first glance to be a mistake, allowing you to amble into a room, shake hands, sit yourself down comfortably in a chair, and exude an easy nonchalance?

Jeff's case history provides some of the answers. He first presented to my clinic in his early 40s. The referring neurologist had become concerned about his patient's tendency to repeat the same questions, the answers clearly eluding him. Jeff was single, lived with an elderly mother, and remarkably, was still employed part time as a college lecturer. His subject was post-Napoleonic France, 1814 to 1850, and from the way he described the course's content to me, it never varied. The subject matter, at least in his hands, had ossified. This was his professional lifeline. He had his set of eight lectures down pat, cemented into his dwindling memory stores. Through a process of repetition over a decade, before his memory began declining, Jeff had gone through the material so many times he was sure he could recite the lectures in his sleep. The information was so thoroughly encoded, all he needed to do was to recite the fixed content with the help of a familiar PowerPoint presentation, now doubling as a memory aid, to his unsuspecting class.

Questions from his students, he acknowledged, presented something more of a challenge and hinted to him that all was not necessarily well with his cognition. But so adept had he become in fudging, obfuscating, and essentially rambling on and on that he filled in the blanks of is answers with verbiage. None of this was deliberate. Not surprisingly, the questions dwindled with time. He put this down to a progressive lack of interest from a younger generation who thought they could find every answer on the internet. This rationalization sustained him. All was well in his world.

The part-time work never troubled him either. There were no money worries. "My mother is worth a pile," he blurted out to me one day. When I suggested she should come along to one of his future appointments, he fixed me with an odd look and demanded to know why. "To help plan for the future," I suggested. Unable to look inwards, unaware of the full extent of his impaired memory and buoyed by his ability to keep teaching, the thought of having his elderly mother become involved in his future care left Jeff incredulous. He stopped coming to see me. Telephone calls and letters offering an appointment were ignored.

Four years passed and then one day his name resurfaced, quite unexpectedly, in an email from his general practitioner, who wanted his patient reassessed. The passage of time had done little to change Jeff's appearance. He perhaps looked a little frailer than when I had last seen him, but observing him walk around and engage superficially with other patients in the waiting area outside my office one would never have known he had MS without access to his medical notes. To my surprise, he was still teaching the same eight-lecture course. The one big change in the interim, however, had been the death of his mother. He had inherited the "pile" as sole heir, and before long it had shrunk to a fraction. Aghast, I asked where it had all gone. In reply, he rummaged in his wallet and pulled out a picture of his wife, who immediately brought to mind Raymond Chandler's memorable line, "[She] was a blonde. A blonde to make a bishop kick a hole in a stained-glass window." The predatory marriage had, of course, been brief, and now he was bereft. Not at his squandered fortune, mind you, but rather in response to his other loss, the love of his life. Oh, how he missed her. He pined for her. This was why he had come back to see me. Could I provide some couples counseling, he wanted to know.

When it comes to treating MS-related memory impairment, a systematic review has concluded that an array of medications including disease-modifying therapies, memory-enhancing drugs, such as donepezil hydrochloride and rivastigmine, and putative memory boosters, such as ginkgo biloba, are ineffective.[41] However, results from cognitive rehabilitation, where much of the focus has been on memory, are promising. A couple of studies have targeted working memory by designing interventions geared toward improving performance on the n-back task. In one of these studies, 29 people with MS and 29 healthy participants were randomly split into treatment and nontreatment groups, with the former undergoing adaptive n-back training for 60 minutes a day over four days. The results revealed that those individuals, both with and without MS, who received the training responded quicker and obtained more correct responses on the 2-back and 3-back versions of the test. These positive changes were accompanied by a decrease in brain activation noted on functional MRI recorded while participants were completing the postintervention assessments.[42] A similar result, but this time with electrophysiological confirmatory correlates, has been reported by Covey et al.,[43] who administered 20 sessions of n-back training to 12 people with MS and 12 people without. Following the interventions, improvements were noted not only on the 3-back but also on indices of processing speed, complex attention, and reasoning ability. The cognitive benefits accrued were accompanied by improved evoked potential indices. These findings mirror those obtained on functional MRI (fMRI)[42] and speak to the presence of brain plasticity, the modifiable nature of brain function in response to a therapeutic intervention.

Given the dysfunctional nature of encoding and consolidation in people with MS, it follows that a number of memory rehabilitation studies have focused on these processes. The Story Memory Technique was designed to enhance new learning by utilizing context and imagery. One study utilized this intervention in a double-blind placebo-controlled randomized clinical trial of 86 people with MS.[14] The placebo intervention entailed the person with MS meeting and taking part in non-training-oriented activities. All interventions were given twice a week over five weeks. All participants underwent neuropsychological testing prior to the interventions, immediately after them, and then again after six months. The results revealed that those individuals who received the memory training were better able to learn new material, an improvement that was maintained by six months postintervention. In addition, other positive changes came with improved memory, such as enhanced general contentment and, according to informants, less apathy and better executive functioning. In a subsequent study, the authors confined their sample selection to people with progressive MS only and achieved the same result.[44] Functional brain imaging once again provides the mechanistic explanation for the intervention's effectiveness. A comparison of pre- and postintervention fMRI data revealed a reduction in brain activation in those networks involved in new learning.[45] As with the imaging data from the working memory rehabilitation trials, reduced activation postintervention indicates a brain working more efficiently.

A different memory rehabilitation approach is the Strategy-based Training to Enhance Memory (STEM) treatment. This entails teaching the individual three distinct, complementary memory strategies, each with its own proven efficacy. Self-generation is based on the principle that information that is self-generated is better remembered than provided information. The second principle is spaced learning, which takes as its premise that new learning is improved when new information is spaced over time rather than given as consecutive learning trials. The third component to STEM is practice retrieval, which is based on data showing that self-testing (e.g., quizzing) leads to better retrieval than restudying information multiple times. The results of an eight-session double-blind placebo-controlled pilot study utilizing STEM in a small sample of people with MS revealed benefits in self-report measures of daily functioning.[46] While comparisons between neuropsychological performance pre- and post-testing fell just short of statistical significance, the effect size (a more meaningful marker of between-group differences) was moderate to large, supporting the efficacy of the intervention.

The positive results reported here are offset to a degree by a study that failed to find any cognitive benefits from the rehabilitation provided.[47] This result was not surprising, however, for the primary aim of the study was on learning to cope with cognitive problems, a limitation noted by the authors. In addition, no enduring improvement in quality of life was found with rehabilitation even though the intervention did lead to less subjective memory complaints. Notwithstanding some notable successes to date, a Cochrane Review that predates the arrival of computerized interventions provides lukewarm support for the benefits of memory rehabilitation, citing numerous methodological limitations in the studies completed thus far. These include enrolling subjects with mild or no deficits to begin with, interventions that are not tailored to the deficits present, too few intervention sessions, and a dearth of data that confirms improvements in real-world functioning.[48]

The studies referenced so far rely on research assistants to administer the interventions. As with the administration of neuropsychological testing, limited resources can be a major determinant as to who gets treated or not. Once more, computers potentially provide a way around the resource hurdle. One such program is RehaCom, which contains rehabilitation modules for memory, attention, and executive functioning. This allows the therapist to choose the module(s) to match the person's deficits. The evidence in terms of memory rehabilitation is encouraging, with benefits accruing after 10 sessions given over five weeks.[49] Most impressive are the results from a RehaCom trial for people with secondary progressive MS (SPMS) that was administered in their homes.[50] In a randomized, sham-controlled trial, 26 people with SPMS were divided into treatment and control groups. Those in the active (RehaCom) group were given 24 sessions of 45 minutes each over an eight-week period entirely at home. The control group was asked to complete nonspecific computer-based activities at the same frequency and duration over the course of eight weeks. The benefits of RehaCom were apparent not only for memory but also for processing speed, fatigue, depression, and overall quality of life.

RehaCom is one of a number of similar computerized cognitive-training programs now commercially available. The consensus is that they are effective with respect to overall and specific indices of cognition, but more data are needed on the other potential benefits that might accompany cognitive improvement—for example, to quality of life, mood, and most importantly, real-world functioning.[51]

The rehabilitation approaches outlined above share one thing in common irrespective of their method of delivery. They are all designed to improve cognition, at best, or failing that, halt further decline. While these remedial approaches potentially offer the memory-impaired person with MS the best treatment options, there is another approach to rehabilitation that helps those with impairment compensate for their deficits. These compensatory strategies will not bring about an improvement in memory or other aspects of cognition, but they can assist the individual in mitigating the effects of the impairment. Here the key strategies are planning, practice, repetition, and routine, which can bolster residual abilities. Having the forgetful person write out a daily agenda and then ensuring that the person checks it regularly is one way to lessen the chance of appointments being missed or tasks overlooked. Incorporating technology into this structure and routine can be helpful too.

NeuroPage is one such memory aid that has proven effective. This program sends reminder messages to mobile phones at prearranged times. Given the ubiquitous presence of mobile devices, the reach of such an intervention is vast. A multicenter, randomized controlled crossover trial has confirmed the benefits of this approach.[52] Compared to a control intervention in which people with MS were phoned at similar intervals but given news updates and sports scores, the reminder messages significantly reduced the number of daily diary items forgotten, and this came with a significant lessening in psychological distress.

Compensatory and remedial strategies are complementary and ideally both should be offered in a clinical setting. The availability of resources, however, dictates that the latter may be hard to find, whereas the former should be available to everyone.

FIVE

Planning and Problem Solving

EXECUTIVE FUNCTION REFERS to the brain's ability to make decisions and solve problems using the building blocks of planning and sequencing while retaining a necessary degree of flexibility that in the most effective of problem solvers includes the ability to think in the abstract, when required. It also encompasses attention, inhibitory control, and working memory, the latter referring to limited amounts of information held temporarily online, as it were, by the brain for this very purpose. It is therefore helpful to view executive function as a top-down mental process, its role akin to that of a conductor in a large symphony orchestra—that central, pivotal entity that directs, incorporates, discards, manipulates, and ultimately synthesizes a constellation of smaller discrete components to produce the desired effect. This might be the glorious sounds of a Beethoven symphony in the case of our maestro or, coming back to cognition, the solution to problems that range from the mundane to the complex and which determine how effectively we navigate the challenges and vicissitudes of everyday living.

When executive function falters, life understandably becomes more demanding. The case history of a patient of mine who loves to bake cakes illustrates this very well. Sally is not a baker by occupation. She works in the accounts receivable department of a large importer. Her job requires little flexibility. In principle, the accounts go out and the cash comes in, the outgoings and incomings matching one another. When they don't, she hands the file off to a different department, to people of a harder temperament, who make the difficult phone calls. Sally has done this work for 20 years. Part of the office furniture is how she sees herself. Blessed with a cheery dispossession, she has a friendly hello for everyone despite her neuropathic pain, which hobbles her gait, the most prominent of her visible signs of multiple sclerosis. But there is another disability hidden from view that is slowly, stealthily, inexorably eroding her quality of life.

Sally must work. There is a mortgage to pay, and her husband is off with a bad back after an industrial accident crushed a few vertebrae and left him with a lot of pain and a taste for opiates. They have no children, and Sally has come to accept that, although the heartache lingers. The formulaic nature of what she does in the office, which never deviates from a set routine, allows her to get the job finished. Nine to five, match the in and out columns, and her work is done. Twenty years of repetition, which in Sally's case is perfect because her executive dysfunction is her real Achilles' heel, not the limp. Repetition, structure, routine—this is the Holy Trinity that gets her through each day at work. Ask her to think outside the box, give her a new set of tasks, change the system, or introduce novelty and her job would be in jeopardy, never mind the sunny temperament, two decades of experience, and unwavering company loyalty. "If it ain't broke, then don't fix it," is how her boss often begins one of his little homilies that he is so fond of, and thank goodness for that because it is keeping her in a job.

Where things start falling apart is not in the office but at home, with her baking. Ever since childhood Sally has loved to bake. Her mother had been a fine baker too, and it was from her that Sally learned the basic skills that she would hone later as an adult. She was the youngest of five children, the only girl, and she recalls the joy of that first Saturday afternoon of each month in the kitchen with her mother, surrounded by all the paraphernalia that would be used to turn eggs and milk and flour into something so beautiful and scrumptious that the whole process seemed like a conjurer's trick. She must have been about 5 or 6 years of age when her mother began allowing her to stir the batter in a big silver bowl until it was smooth and creamy, and then the two of them would pour it ever so carefully into the tins that were shaped like hearts, squares, rectangles, and stars. Soon the kitchen would fill with a heavenly smell as they went about preparing the colored icings that would fill the tubes with different nozzles that helped pattern their designs. The afternoon would fly by, and by the time Dad and Sally's brothers came back from the baseball diamond or hockey rink, the cake would be perfectly finished and left for show on the dinner table like some prized trophy, which it was to her, and it seemed such a pity to cut it until that first slice, so light and firm and just the right texture, banished any qualms, and the oohs and aahs of her brothers came like music to her ears.

Sally married young, just out of her two-year business administration program from a local college. And no sooner had she settled in to her apartment than she started baking. Now it was her mother's turn to be the assistant, for it had long been apparent to both that the child had outstripped the parent in this department. The first Saturday of every month was given over to their joint passion, and in keeping with tradition, the finished cake would be left on the dining room table to be admired before it was sliced into generous portions and devoured by family, friends, and neighbors. The apartment was always crowded when cake was on offer.

The happy idyll in the kitchen ended with her mother's sudden death from a heart attack. "Taken away by one too many cakes," one of the mourners was overheard saying. My patient didn't bake for a year after that. The loss was so sudden and painful she could not bring herself to return to an activity that now reduced her to tears. The oven remained cold.

Life moved on. After time off for bereavement, Sally returned to work. The couple, with a little more money in hand, moved into a townhouse, which Sally set about redecorating. She hoped to start a family. She made new friends at work. And it was one of these new friendships that pulled her back into the kitchen to bake. The woman at the workstation next to hers was pregnant, and with the baby due soon, Sally spontaneously offered to bake a cake for the christening. "It just kinda slipped out," she recalled, "and I didn't feel like crying." The cake she baked was a real beauty—a light, tiered chiffon with pale pink icing embellished with a flock of smiling storks that circled a crib. Sally put all her love for her mother into that cake. She could feel her mother's presence at her shoulder every step of the way, and this comforted her. The joy of baking was back.

News of Sally's baking prowess spread quickly around the office. Expectant mothers and parents with young children approached her with requests. She took to photographing her cakes and made a presentation album of them, which made the rounds at work. Soon her weekends were confined to the kitchen. The extra income was a boon, but more than that, she loved what she was doing. As Sally stood in the kitchen working her magic for colleagues and friends, she fantasized about the cakes she would bake for her own children. They would have such fun together, just like old times. But the children never came. Sally and her husband tried everything the fertility clinic suggested, but without success. She wanted to adopt. Her husband didn't, and Sally didn't fight him on it. Instead, she continued to bake for her nieces and nephews and other people's children, taking joy in their excited, shining faces as they ogled their birthday cakes, even as she felt the pangs of her loss.

Such was her success that she began toying with the idea of quitting her office job and opening a cake business. MS put an end to that. The disease-modifying drugs were expensive, and her accounts receivable position, while boring, came with a good benefits package. She never skipped her every-other-day injections, even though they made a mess of her skin. Life was a compromise, she told herself, even if at the moment she was the one making all the compromises. Ten years into their marriage, Sally's husband fell 30 feet from some scaffolding and ruined his back. Now her work became a respite from his chronic pain complaints and constant importuning for more medication. These were dark days for Sally, but she never quit baking. It was a lifeline, something to look forward to on the weekends, a skill that pulled her out, momentarily, from a humdrum, disappointing life and let her connect with people in a way that managing the ledgers never could. Even her husband's lugubrious expression perked up with a cup of tea and a thick slice of her chocolate cake—the cocoa rich and creamy and given a delicious chewiness by thin shavings of a peanut-butter-flavored toffee.

So imagine this woman's distress when her baking, her salvation, started to falter. As she explained it to me, baking involved a lot of meticulous preparation. She had to plan beforehand what she wanted to do. While there was a detailed recipe to follow, she had never felt bound to it, inserting her own little variations into the process, allowing her individuality to find a place in the complex mix of ingredients and instructions. While the process was intuitive, it nevertheless still had to follow certain basic rules and an overall game plan. This necessary flexibility, in which she moved in and out of a set recipe, taking what she wanted from it while discarding aspects she felt limited her, was one of the central features that made baking so much fun. Sally recognized her approach was something of a high-wire act, for there was no safety net to catch her mistakes. You either got it 100% right or else you crashed and burned. There was no middle ground. Mistakes could not be hidden under the icing, and as for a bad icing, well . . . and here she shuddered.

I marveled at the description of what went on in Sally's kitchen on a Saturday afternoon. The process actually started earlier in the day when she set out to purchase the ingredients that were the fuel to her creativity. Once she had what was needed, she would mentally map out the strategy to follow over the next three to four hours. Planning and sequencing were essential here, but in addition to having good organization, Sally had to remain cognitively nimble, for there were always surprises lying in wait when you diverged, even slightly, from the printed page. Going about baking this way made it exciting—a challenge, a voyage of discovery, for if the end point was clearly known in advance, exactly how to get there was not. The journey as much as the cake itself had become the destination.

Now, 15 years after her MS first manifested as a blurry vision in her left eye, Sally's consummate skills as a baker were starting to unravel. To begin with, she was finding it harder to deviate from the recipe. It was one thing to step into uncharted waters but quite another to find her way back, and when this went awry, she would lose her thread and the whole process would unravel. "Don't forget," she reminded me, "time was also of the essence." You had to keep to your timelines. Leave the cake in the oven for too long and it would come out dry and, heaven forbid, even a little burned. On the other hand, rush things along and the cake would emerge too soggy. Which meant you could never take your eye off the clock. So when a problem arose, and this was now happening with increasing frequency, Sally had to solve it under intense time pressure. And it was here that she was finding it difficult to think on her feet. Her mental flexibility was abandoning her. Solutions that would come effortlessly to her a year back were now harder to find. By the time she had worked out what to do, the cake was ruined.

Sally's response to this crisis in the kitchen was to step back from her creativity and stick closer to the recipe. But even here she was running into problems. The sequencing that was so necessary to a successful outcome was also proving elusive. On occasion, she would mix-up the order of what was required, and whereas in the past this would not have proved disastrous, now she lacked the mental agility to bounce back and work around the roadblock. The frustrating part, she explained to me, was that she could see where she was going wrong, but she could not find the solution in time to correct the mistake. Moreover, and this troubled her greatly, she kept making the same mistakes over and over, unable to find her way out of the morass until, in frustration and on the verge of tears, she would scoop up the whole mess and dump it in the garbage feeling devastated. It took all her willpower just to wash the utensils and clean her kitchen after that. Five o'clock on a Saturday afternoon arrived, and there was no longer a show cake on the dining room table and a delicious aroma in the house. The kitchen was dark, cold, and silent now. A large part of her life, stretching back to childhood, felt alarmingly out of reach.

To understand why baking a cake, albeit an intricate one, was now presenting an insurmountable problem to an intelligent woman a couple of years shy of her 40th birthday, let us look closely at her performance on a particular cognitive task, the Wisconsin Card Sorting Test (WCST). The test as we know it today dates back to the work of psychologists Myra Gable, Harry Harlow, and David Grant and the latter's master's student, Esther Berg, at the University of Wisconsin in 1945, and it is regarded as a measure of a person's ability to work out concepts and apply a strategy to modify responses to changing conditions.[1] Today, there are different ways this test can be administered, with most testers using a computerized version because it makes the scoring much easier. In the original test, participants are seated before four stimulus cards. They are then given a stack of cards and a simple instruction: sort the cards in a way that matches the four stimulus cards. They are purposely not told what the matching should entail and instead are left to work this out themselves. We can see in figure 5.1 that the cards can be matched by the number (1, 2, 3, 4), color (red, green, blue, yellow), or shape (circle, star, triangle, cross) of the symbols. From the example provided, the card containing the two blue triangles could therefore be matched by

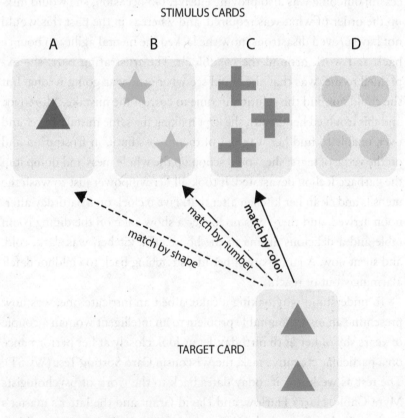

Figure 5.1. The Wisconsin Card Sorting Test

"two" or "blue" or "triangle." The participants will be told "correct" or "incorrect" depending on whether they have worked out the sorting principle. But then the task gets sneaky. After a run of trials, the sorting principle, which may have been a color to start with, is changed without telling the participants. They will now have to shift to a different sort category, say shapes or numbers, and so the test proceeds for a certain number of trials before the sorting code is changed yet again without warning. The inability of participants to make the necessary shifts in a timely fashion will show up as a string of answers that are consistently incorrect. This rigidity of response is termed "perseverative."[2] The number of perseverations is tallied and becomes one of the markers of performance. Other performance indices include the number of categories obtained (the maximum is four) and the number of correct attempts made. The full version of the test contains 256 cards; a shorter version of 128 cards is also available.

Sally started the test well, sorting the cards according to shapes, but when it came to the first shift, she was slow to pick up on it, seemingly stuck (or perseverating, to use the correct neuropsychological jargon) on shapes as her only category. Eventually, in response to repeatedly being told her answers were incorrect, she stopped responding and took a long time to decide what to do next. After choosing colors as her second category, she demonstrated the same perseverative tendency when it came to the next shift, and so the test played out over the 128 trials. Her relative inability to grasp the concepts needed to complete the test smoothly and quickly, her labored responses to each required shift in strategy, and the viscosity of her thinking, as shown by the high number of perseverations, laid bare the dysfunctional nature of her executive functioning. Her days of making elaborate, exquisitely detailed cakes were over. Cognitive abilities, however, lie along a continuum. Sally's executive functions were not ablated. There was still enough residual capacity to make a simpler cake. Her apple crumble remained delicious, that I can personally attest to for she never failed to bring me one, still warm, as a Christmas gift. But once you have scaled the heights and sampled the air on high, being forced to descend and lower your sights can be difficult. That she managed this come down with good grace and a wistful smile spoke volumes to a fine temperament. Which is not to say it didn't hurt.

There are numerous studies going back 30 years showing that people with MS perform more poorly on the WCST than healthy individuals.[3–5] Other card sorting tests of executive function that incorporate the basic principles of the WCST, such as the California Card Sorting Test[6] and the Delis-Kaplan Executive Function System (D-KEFS),[7] have given similar results. The latter was selected by a group of neuropsychologists with a particular expertise in MS research as the flagship executive measure for the Minimal Assessment of Cognitive Function in MS (MACFIMS) battery, a consensus-derived set of cognitive tasks for people with MS.[8] The reason for choosing it over the WCST is the availability of parallel forms of the test, necessary for serial testing to minimize the confounding effects of practice. The WCST, on the other hand, has only a single form.

A third frequently used index of executive dysfunction, one that has worked its way into popular culture, is the Stroop Test.[9] Given that individuals can read words faster than they can identify and name colors, merging these discordant abilities into one test challenges an individual's processing speed and selective attention. There are many variations on the Stroop theme, but in one classic version, a person is presented with a list of 24 words naming four colors: red, blue, yellow, and green. These words are written in white on a black background and repeated in four rows of six words each across a computer screen. The individual is asked to read the name of the colors from left to right as quickly as possible and the task is timed. In the next paradigm, squares of red, blue, yellow, and green replace the words, and the individual has to identify and name each color as quickly as possible. Once more, the test is timed. The two paradigms presented so far are control tasks to record reading and color-identification times. They are the prelude to the full Stroop Test, in which the names of colors are presented in different colors (figure 5.2). The individual is instructed to name the *color* the word is written in, not to read the word itself. Looking at figure 5.2, we can see that while the first word is "blue," the correct answer is yellow. This

BLUE	YELLOW	RED	BLUE	GREEN	RED
GREEN	RED	BLUE	RED	YELLOW	GREEN
YELLOW	BLUE	GREEN	YELLOW	RED	BLUE
RED	GREEN	YELLOW	GREEN	BLUE	YELLOW

Figure 5.2. The Stroop Test

task is also timed. Numerous studies attest to the difficulties people with MS have with the test.[10-13]

Another approach to testing for executive deficits had researchers administer the D-KEFS and the Weekly Calendar Planning Activity to 62 people with MS (of whom, 21 were cognitively impaired) and 38 healthy people.[14] Results were compared to everyday functional performance measured by Actual Reality, a performance-based assessment that entails the use of the internet to undertake real, everyday life activities. The findings showed that the cognitively compromised MS sample performed significantly more poorly on the D-KEFS and Calendar Planning tasks. The Weekly Calendar Planning Activity, in turn, was able to predict performance on most of the Actual Reality tasks. The significance of this study lies in the ecological validity, or real-world relevance, of the data, for it underscores the importance of planning and problem solving to everyday functioning.

We have seen previously how slowed processing speed negatively affects memory. There is evidence it may also influence executive functioning. Data supporting this comes from a study of 50 people with MS and 28 healthy participants who were administered tests of executive function with and without a processing speed element.[15] The MS group performed more poorly than the control group on speeded tasks of executive function. Significantly, after the researchers statistically controlled for these group differences in processing speed, the group differences in executive function disappeared. The conclusion was that slowed processing speed contributed to executive deficits just as it did to other aspects of impaired cognition. While others have reported similar findings,[16] a cautionary note against attributing most executive difficulties to a fall-off in processing speed has been sounded.[17]

Executive function, in turn, influences prospective memory. The latter refers to a form of memory that involves remembering to perform a planned action or recalling a planned intention at some future point in time. We frequently call on it in our daily lives, which makes the dearth of prospective memory research in people with MS surprising. In a study of 39 people with MS and 18 healthy participants, a prospective memory task linking cues with actions was devised and administered together with a wide-ranging battery of standard neuropsychological tests for memory, attention, processing speed, and executive function. Among the latter were two indices from the D-KEFS.[18] To summarize the methodology, the prospective memory task started with participants having to memorize four words or prospective cues (pills, clock, money, apple), each associated with a specific action. The link between the cue and the action was then manipulated so that two of the cue-action pairs were related ("pills" with opening a pillbox and "clock" with telling the examiner the time) and two were not ("money" with watering a plant and "apple" with giving the keys back to the examiner). Participants were provided with the four objects (pillbox, clock, watering can, and keys) and then presented with the cue words (verbally and on a computer screen) embedded in a series of words and nonwords. On detecting the cue word, participants had to perform the action associated with the word. The results revealed numerous cognitive deficits in people with MS, including those for prospective memory. However, it was those individuals with executive impairments who had the greatest difficulty with prospective memory, particularly when it came to completing the appropriate action unrelated to the cue. Of note is that retrospective memory was found to have little impact on prospective memory.

Planning, sequencing, and thinking creatively, the building blocks of executive function, are pivotal in decision making. They help us find solutions to problems, and for the person with MS they are important in successfully adapting and adjusting to the reality of living with a disease that often proves disabling and for which there is no cure. There is evidence that coping mechanisms are integral to these associations. For example, data show that well-preserved executive function can lessen the negative fallout from prominent maladaptive coping strategies.[19] This has implications for rehabilitation in that people with MS who have executive challenges would potentially benefit from less cognitively demanding adaptive coping strategies.

Executive function is one of many factors that can influence the ability to cope. Others may include personality, depression, fatigue, and anxiety. The complexities of these interactions were illustrated in a study that failed to find an association between executive dysfunction and quality of life, a result that at first glance seems surprising.[20] Instead, what the researchers found were more circumscribed relationships, such as non-time-dependent planning correlating with depression, while severity of stress was predicted by a working memory test. Results like these need replication. What is clearer, however, is the bidirectional nature of these associations. In a couple of studies, Arnett et al.[21,22] showed how depression could lead to an impairment in executive function, a result that has been replicated but with an important caveat: depression-induced cognitive dysfunction was confined to those people with more serious, clinically significant depression.[23]

Historically, executive abilities were linked to the functional integrity of the frontal lobes, or to be more precise, a frontal region known as the dorsolateral prefrontal cortex. Milner, in her 1963 landmark study, "Effects of Different Brain Lesions on Card Sorting: The Role of the Frontal Lobes," noted the anatomical link with poor performance on the WCST.[2] Findings from people with MS subsequently reported associations with brain pathology too.[24] Fifty years after Esther Berg completed her master's dissertation on the WCST at the University of Wisconsin, Peter Arnett and colleagues at the same institution showed that poor performance on the test correlated significantly with a heavy frontal lesion load as seen on MRI.[25] Other researchers, far removed from Wisconsin, confirmed the importance of frontal pathology utilizing tests of executive function other than the WCST, most notable the Stroop Test and a spatial planning task based on the Tower of London test.[26] However, increasingly sophisticated brain imaging analyses were starting to show that attributing specific cognitive abnormalities solely to focal brain pathology in people with MS was missing a bigger, more complex picture.

Sally's brain MRI illustrates the point. Her poor performance on the WCST was expected. But a detailed analysis of her brain MRI showed little involvement of the dorsolateral prefrontal cortex. This, too, was not surprising, for we now know that cognition is the product of neural networks connecting dispersed brain regions. The dorsolateral prefrontal cortex is an important region in executive function, as Milner correctly noted, but it is not the only one. In an *Archives of Neurology* article in 2003, Jeff Cummings provided a succinct summary of these discrete, yet interconnected prefrontal-subcortical connections. The *dorsolateral* prefrontal cortex is richly connected to the dorsolateral aspect of the caudate nucleus, the lateral dorsomedial nucleus of the globus pallidus, and the medial dorsal and ventral anterior nuclei of the thalamus.[27] A lesion anywhere within this network, or more likely multifocal damage to the white and gray matter impinging on these tracts, could in theory disrupt or *disconnect* executive abilities. Given that MS is a multifocal disease with lesions and atrophy affecting widely dispersed brain regions, a person with MS might show signs of inflexible problem solving, perseverative responses, and an inability to think abstractly *without* direct involvement of the dorsolateral prefrontal cortex. So it was with Sally, whose baking skills were slipping away from her.

The idea of dysfunction arising from disconnected specialized brain regions can be traced back to the nineteenth century, but it was given fresh impetus by Norman Geschwind in his two-part 1965 publication in *Brain* entitled "Disconnexion Syndromes in Animals and Man."[28] Geschwind's ideas defined behavioral neurology for decades afterward. Published only two years after Milner's important paper, Geschwind's work provided a cogent framework for understanding how circumscribed cognitive deficit like executive dysfunction could arise from such widely dispersed brain abnormalities. Fast forward 50 years and Geschwind's reputation may have lost none of its luster but his theory has, for advances in neuroscience show that disconnection, while still considered relevant, is only part of a more complex picture that now includes the possibility of hyperconnection as a source of cognitive dysfunction.[29]

The current MRI literature pertaining to executive dysfunction in people with MS confirms these theoretical underpinnings. While the brain regions associated with executive dysfunction vary to a degree according to the test of executive function used, the following findings hold true: deficits have been linked to total lesion area; predominantly frontal lesion volume; frontal, parietal, and temporal lesion volume; various markers of brain atrophy, be they global or regional; and indices derived from normal-appearing gray and white matter using diffusion tensor imaging (for a review see Roman and Arnett[17]). These structural brain changes are complemented by a burgeoning functional MRI literature that has revealed asynchrony in networks involving the dorsolateral prefrontal cortex in executive function,[30] the importance of thalamic activation in frontoparietal networks associated with processing speed in executive function,[31] and differences in connectivity according to disease course.[32]

The consequences of executive difficulties are graphically illustrated in Sally's case history. Their reach, however, extends well beyond the kitchen. Sally was able to maintain her work so long because the nature of what she did remain unchanged. A set routine was manageable because the cognitive skills necessary for her work did not demand mental flexibility, problem solving, thinking out the box, or planning. Speed of response was important, but Sally's job requirements had been drilled into her decades back when her ability to learn something new had been robustly intact. Her work skills were by now hardwired through endless repetition—she could do the job in her sleep was how she viewed things. Arrive at work the same time each morning, switch on the computer, adjust the air conditioner, check the inbox, feed the invoices into a document collector that automatically read the content, which then appeared on her screen, push another button for a software program to populate the blank fields with the content of the document, give it all a quick once over to make sure the automated process had covered all the angles (which it always did given that it was 100% reliable), push another button to endorse payment, wait for the confirmation of payment to appear, print the proof of payment document, file the online copy (which the program did by default anyway), and then you were on to the next item. Take a midmorning coffee break—not decaffeinated because she needed the energy pick-me-up—and then back to the same routine until lunch. An afternoon caffeine boost around three o'clock, then the homestretch that took her to the five o'clock knockoff time. Monday through Friday, day in, day out, Dependable Sally could be found at her station making sure the payments were processed on time, her efficiency honed by endless repetition—way beyond the 10,000 hours considered by Malcolm Gladwell as the key to success in any field of endeavor—and smoothly, too, like one of her batters—which is where the analogy ended because her job was the antithesis of what she did in the kitchen with her gleaming stand mixer and assorted high-end attachments.

However, "life," as Samuel Butler remarked, "is like giving a concert on the violin while learning to play the instrument." One needs to learn and adapt quickly and not repeat the same mistakes. When cognition starts declining and executive functions unravel, the ramifications can be profound. Managing one's finances can become challenging. Financial capacity, the ability to take care of one's financial affairs in a way that is consistent with one's personal self-interest and long-standing values, can be undermined. People with MS are vulnerable here, with data showing that financial capacity may be impaired in up to 50% of those with progressive forms of the disease.[33] Impaired cognition is the culprit—in particular, deficits in executive function and working memory.[34] Other negative financial implications may follow too. A two-year longitudinal study of factors affecting employment in 124 people with relapsing-remitting MS showed that executive difficulties, alone among other cognitive deficits, and physical disability were the two factors that predicted a falloff in employment status.[35] A systematic review of the topic of employment in people with MS confirmed the importance of intact executive function, among other cognitive abilities, in keeping a job.[36]

Given the real-world implications of executive dysfunction, and of impaired cognition in general, attention is increasingly shifting to management strategies. Similar to what was noted earlier in relation to abnormalities in processing speed and memory, a recent systematic review[37] found no compelling evidence of medication-related benefits for executive dysfunction, be it from disease-modifying therapies or symptomatic treatments. A more optimistic picture is, however, to be found with cognitive rehabilitation, although it is notable that considerably less attention has been devoted to executive difficulties than to memory, in particular, and processing speed abnormalities. In a small six-week placebo-controlled randomized trial, researchers divided 40 people with MS into three groups: those receiving cognitive rehabilitation, placebo intervention, and no intervention at all.[38] The content of the intervention was not made clear, with the researchers simply referring to "textbook exercises for executive training." Be that as it may, the active treatment group showed statistically significant gains in executive function and verbal learning compared to the other two groups. Further, albeit partial, support comes from a study of 120 inpatients with MS who were randomly assigned to multidisciplinary rehabilitation groups with and without a cognitive intervention component.[39] The cognitive intervention was geared toward attaining goals for coping with cognitive difficulties. Four weeks of rehabilitation were given to both groups followed by three months of biweekly telephone calls focusing on goal attainment for the cognitive intervention group only. Similar improvements in executive functioning were found in both groups, but only those in the cognitive rehabilitation group reported improved emotional well-being. At first glance, the cognitive result may seem surprising. One possible explanation, postulated by the research team, related to patients in the general rehabilitation program having been given lectures on cognitive and psychological aspects of MS, as well as options for sessions with a psychologist. This, in turn, could have instilled in them an awareness of the importance of executive functioning and coping strategies for managing the challenges of everyday life. Whether this translated into the control group setting their own goals is not known. What is clear, however, even if the mechanism is not, is that executive difficulties are to a degree remediable.

A computer-assisted cognitive rehabilitation intervention confirms this. In a multicenter, randomized, controlled trial limited to people with relapsing-remitting MS with mild to moderate cognitive impairment, 58 people with MS were randomly assigned to receive either RehaCom or standard clinical care that lacked a cognitive component.[40] Ten weeks of treatment led to significant improvements in attention, speed of information processing, verbal and visuospatial memory, and executive function, but only in the RehaCom group. While improvement was maintained for six months postintervention, this was limited to attention only.

Finally, before concluding this chapter on executive function and, in doing so, bringing the sections on cognitive dysfunction to an end, mention must be made of exercise as a putative intervention for global and domain-specific impairments. The theory goes that regular exercise, which has an anti-inflammatory effect, enhances neurogenesis, which in turn promotes the production of brain-derived neurotrophic factor, all of which may help cognition. Cognitive benefits following exercise have been reported in older adults who are healthy,[41,42] have mild cognitive impairment,[43,44] or have Alzheimer's disease.[45,46] Similar effects may also accrue in other neurological conditions, such as stroke[47] and traumatic brain injury,[48] and major mental illness, such as schizophrenia.[49] A consistent thread that runs through all the systematic reviews cited here is a concern about methodological limitations, the presence of which dilutes the strength of the conclusions.

This concern permeates the MS exercise literature as well. Despite a couple of studies reporting modest effect sizes,[50,51] a systematic review and multilevel meta-analysis of 13 clinical trials revealed no overall positive effects on cognition, be it global or domain specific.[52] The majority of interventions prescribed aerobic exercise alone (n=8) or in combination with resistance training (n=4), and there was a single resistance-training study. The major shortcomings that cloud the findings include, among others, failure to exclude cognitively intact individuals, the absence of validated neuropsychological batteries known to be sensitive to deficits in this population, and a failure to report sample power calculations, intention to treat analyses, and adverse events, including specific dropout rates. The authors noted that the volume of exercise prescribed accounted for an important percentage of within and between study heterogeneity. This opens the door to the possibility of a higher training dose exerting a small effect on global cognitive improvement.

While further work exploring the benefits of exercise is needed, one potentially effective approach entails combining exercise with another intervention that improves cognition, namely, cognitive rehabilitation, with the aim of assessing whether there is a synergistic effect between the two treatments.[53,54] The results from a preliminary study give cause for cautious optimism.[55]

SIX

Global Impairment and the Unraveling of Personality

IN ALL THE case histories described so far, I have described individuals whose impaired cognition was largely, but not exclusively, confined to a single domain, be it processing speed, memory, or executive function. I did this because relatively isolated deficits make it easier to explain the particular challenges that accompany them. However, people with multiple sclerosis frequently display numerous cognitive deficits.

As noted previously, cognitive impairment is determined relative to data obtained from healthy people matched for age, sex, and years of education. Thresholds for impairment are determined statistically, and one widely used approach is to base impairment on a score that falls 1.5 standard deviations below mean or average normative scores. Should a person with MS fail two or more indices of cognition in this manner— for example, processing speed and memory—then that person is deemed by convention to be globally impaired. The cognitive impairment rates of 40%, 80%, and 90% in people with relapsing-remitting, primary progressive, and secondary progressive MS, respectively, refer to global impairment.[1]

Specific, relatively isolated cognitive deficits can come with functional limitations, as the case histories given thus far reveal. However, people with MS who are globally impaired face even greater challenges in their day-to-day functioning. As the deficits stack up, the functional impairments increase. In situations like these, the cognitive deficits are often part of a clinical picture in which there is more extensive neurological compromise. The cumulative effects on the individual and her family can be devastating, as the following case history reveals.

Emma is in her early 50s and has been referred to me because of cognitive concerns. She uses a walker to ambulate at home. When away from home, she uses a power wheelchair. She used to work as a cosmetic salesperson but stopped 10 years back when it became increasingly difficult for her to stand for prolonged periods. She is married with a grown son who works but still lives at home. Her husband works night shifts as a security guard. He chose the night work so that he could keep an eye on his wife during the day. When he is at work, their son looks in on his mom.

Within minutes of meeting Emma, I see in stark focus the magnitude of what she and her family face. A decade of sedentary living has left a mark. She appears overweight, disheveled. Gone is the chic salesperson. Not a splash of makeup now, hair hacked short, wearing a stained and rumpled tracksuit. The only aspect of clothing that is clean are her shoes—a pair of sneakers, spotlessly white with pristine Velcro straps and tread intact, no signs of wear and tear. The footwear of disabled people often tells a poignant story. Shoes are worn but never used. Shoes that are years old look like they have just come out of the box. The one item of clothing most likely to get scuffed and roughed up by grimy floors, filthy sidewalks, and muddy pathways—the only item of clothing that is constantly in contact with dirt—and yet always looks immaculate. A telltale sign of a life curtailed.

Emma sits heavily in her wheelchair, indifferent to the interview. She has no idea why she has been brought to see me. It does not concern her. I ask whether she would like to transfer to a chair. She shrugs. "It's all the same to me," she replies. There is not a spark of curiosity about the proceedings. She denies feeling depressed. She gives me permission to speak with her husband, Bob, who is in the waiting room.

Bob is a large man, still in his night shift uniform with faux-sergeant epaulets and a thick canvas belt that is home to an enormous bunch of keys and an astonishing array of devices, including a walkie-talkie with flapping aerial, a pager, two flashlights small and large, a collapsible truncheon, an assortment of screwdrivers, and other items that defy easy recognition. He is clearly very stressed. He gives a history that is all too familiar in an MS clinic. The couple has been together for 25 years. The early years were happy, he was making good money in secure jobs, their son was born, and in their spare time they decorated their suburban home. All their aspirations were being met in a respectable neighborhood where every family had two cars in the driveway, a neatly clipped lawn, and a future that offered stability and financial security. Emma's diagnosis of MS, while a shock to begin with, didn't really alter the flow of life. She remained relatively well for years, and the family continued to prosper.

Ten years back, however, things started to change. Emma's walking faltered, her fatigue became overwhelming, and bit by bit, her level of functioning began slipping. Activities that had been taken for granted and thoroughly enjoyed were given up, one by one. Gone was the Sunday morning walk, the monthly dinner party for friends, the cross-country skiing, the charity work for the local church. The world starting closing in on them as a lifestyle once active and fulfilling shrank. The process was slow but inexorable and marked by two Rubicons that had to be crossed. The first was the use of a cane, the second the purchase of a power wheelchair. Each was strongly resisted at first, as if a refusal to accept these markers of disability would somehow keep the illness at bay. Acknowledging their need had been hard for Emma, her acceptance ultimately forced by necessity. To be sure, it had been tough on Bob to see his wife's faltering gait, perpetual tiredness, and stumbles and falls. But what had been harder by far was to see and live with a partner whose cognition was failing. As he explained to me, navigating transfers from house to car and from bed to walker, or providing help when it came to dressing or showering, demanded a big adjustment. But these had been made with the assistance of personal support workers and a realization from all involved that an increasingly constrained life would now move slower, more cautiously. A truncated lifestyle still left the door open to enjoying a movie together, sharing a lovely meal in a new restaurant, even going on a cruise where there were facilities and help for the disabled. Escalating cognitive difficulties, however, closed this off these avenues of respite. How could a movie be enjoyed when it was not remembered? How was one to take pleasure from a restaurant when the choice of a varied menu induced confusion? What pleasure was there in a cruise when an unfamiliar environment triggered panic? Gradually, these activities fell away until all that was left were days at home spent in dull silence, conversation stilled, Bob's marital role reduced to that of caregiver to a person he still loved. What sustained him now were the memories of bygone days, of a vibrant woman, who every now and then still peeked out of the shell of a person that MS had reduced her to.

Neuropsychological testing confirmed my clinical impression of profound cognitive compromise. Processing speed, learning, memory, and executive functioning were significantly impaired. In addition, Emma's lack of interest in, and enthusiasm and concern for, all aspects of her life was indicative of a marked degree of apathy. This indifference, which made her engagement in cognitive rehabilitation impossible, proved resistant to a succession of psychostimulant medications, such as methylphenidate, modafinil, amantadine, and assorted amphetamine derivatives. As a last throw of the psychotropic dice, I gave her a trial of the memory-enhancing drug used in people with Alzheimer's disease, donepezil hydrochloride. In 2004, there had been a flurry of excitement in the MS world when a paper was published in *Neurology*, the flagship journal of the American Academy of Neurology, showing that donepezil (trade name Aricept) could improve memory in people with MS.[2] The problem with the study, however, was its limited sample size. A follow-up multicenter study powered appropriately this time failed to replicate the result, and with it the hopes of many people with MS who had advanced cognitive dysfunction faded.[3] Still, giving the drug to Emma was worth a try, more so as another small MS study limited to residents of nursing homes and assisted-living facilities showed that abnormal behaviors, including apathy, could improve after as little as four weeks of treatment.[4] Bob, who by now had become Emma's substitute decision maker, was all for the medication even if Emma appeared indifferent to it. Six months of treatment at a therapeutic dose made not one bit of difference. The drug was discontinued.

The three individual components that make up a person's mental state—cognition, mood, and behavior—lie along a continuum in terms of their expression. With the onset of neurological illness, these three pillars can be affected to differing degrees. Some people with MS may be fortunate and escape change. Others may become cognitively compromised, show mood instability, or display alterations in behavior. The least fortunate, like Emma, are affected across more than one domain.

So what, then, is personality? How is this different from the mental state and its three component parts? Personality has been defined as the distinctive pattern of behavior, including thoughts and emotions, that characterize each individual's adaptation to the situations of his or her life.[5] This, too, can change in response to a brain disease like multiple sclerosis. To better understand how this can come about, let us return to Emma and her devoted husband, Bob.

After a while, Emma stopped coming to see me. There was no point, really. It took a lot of effort on Bob's part to get her ready and into her wheelchair, which then had to be loaded into the family van, now specially modified for this purpose. On snowy days, this was particularly tough to do because the family home did not have a garage, and so the slippery, sludgy pathway from front door to curbside parking had to be navigated. This could prove treacherous, as Emma had lost the ability to navigate her behemoth of a chair and so the task fell once more to her stressed husband, who—encumbered by heavy coat and gloves on a frigid morning—would have to stand in front her and walk slowly backward, guiding the motorized chair as he went. On one occasion, when Emma tried to help, her clumsy movements on the power lever jolted the chair forward and she ran over Bob, leaving him with some nasty cuts and bruises.

The challenge with Emma's appointments, however, was only in part logistic. After the struggle to get her to my office, she would have nothing to say. Bob would remind her of things she had forgotten, to which she responded with either a giggle or a quizzical shrug. Such was her level of cognitive impairment, she now retained very little recent memory or ability to plan tasks, and accompanying this dementia was a change in personality. A profound apathy interspersed with the occasional sharp outburst of irritability had settled over her. Her drive and motivation were gone. Whole days could be spent in her padded wheelchair doing nothing, sitting passively in front of the TV, where she was parked each morning awaiting Bob's return from the nightshift, a return that was greeted with indifference. This apathy was evident during her appointments with me too. She never spontaneously asked a question, initiated conversation, or volunteered an observation. Her symptoms by now were numerous, and yet not a word of complaint came from her. The world was passing her by unnoticed. Even within her home, the comings and goings of Bob and their son were barely acknowledged. Accompanying Emma's cognitive decline was loss of empathy, that ability to detect and sympathize with the distress of others. She was oblivious to the cost her illness was exerting, not only on herself but on her family too. At one appointment, when Bob broke down and began weeping, Emma sat there silently, seemingly unmoved by his racking sobs. It was then that Bob became my patient, and it was agreed that he would attend future appointments without Emma, unless her behavior changed enough to give concern.

Bob needed a person to talk to. He also badly needed some psychoeducation. For what troubled him the most were not the physical demands of caring for his profoundly disabled wife—he had a lot of assistance from community nurses and personal support workers for that—but rather the loss of emotional intimacy. To begin with, he was surprised by Emma's indifference to her illness and the effects it was having on him and their son. This perplexity gave way to hurt. Surely, she could see what a toll her immobility, passiveness, and incapacity were exerting on him, couldn't she? He was by now exhausted and struggling to keep his night job going while attending to his wife during the day, between his naps. He was not looking for a thank you. The smallest hint of endearment would have sufficed, some spontaneous show, even a glimmer, of emotional connection. A little love and affection, that's all—never mind the physical intimacy, because that had long been abandoned. But affection never came, and with her interminable silences, broken occasionally by a word of rebuke, his resentment began.

Now that Bob had a place to vent, one theme came to the surface immediately. On one level, he could understand that MS has taken away Emma's legs, her coordination, and even her continence. But why was she so stubborn and at times nasty? Why could she not do anything to ease his burden? Why was she repeatedly calling out for him during the day even though he had to get some sleep after working all night? Why had she become indifferent to her own son and the challenges he was having with his girlfriend. What kind of mother could behave like this? How on earth could this woman who had once been so loving and generous and outgoing now be so selfish? For selfish is what she had become, he assured me, selfish to the bone. "If she wants something, she wants it now, not later—even if that means waking me up—and then she shouts at me for responding too slowly for her liking!"

Bob was skeptical at first when I explain how advanced MS can affect personality. He had no difficulty grasping the cognitive fallout from MS—his wife's memory loss was readily apparent—but personality change was a more challenging concept for him to accept. This was more personal for him, for he still retained so many fond memories of who Emma had once been. To Bob, his wife's indifference and her episodes of verbal hostility seemed deliberate at times—willful and designed to frustrate and hurt—and the theory that he had formulated to explain it, and which it was my task to debunk, was that Emma was deliberately behaving this way because of her frustrations with her disease and the limitations that came with it. "Doc," confided Bob, "it's almost like her saying, Well, if I'm going down, I'm bloody well going to take everyone with me."

I started by acknowledging his distress. The first few sessions were spent discussing what he needed to do to look after his physical and emotional health. Notwithstanding his anger at his wife, Bob remained devoted to her and taking time away from her on weekends was difficult for him, even though he knew she was being well cared for by a personal support worker in his absence. Multifaceted guilt troubled him greatly: I can walk but she cannot; I can get out the house but she cannot; I can partake in so much of life that is now inaccessible to her; I have not done enough to ease her burden. And most troubling of all, the remorse that underlay his anger with her. At times it made him feel ashamed.

Bit by bit we chipped away at these issues. It helped when I normalized his emotions, let him know that what he felt was shared by other caregivers, that he, too, was allowed to feel frustrated and deflated and exhausted at times, that Emma's MS was a shared burden. I made reference to the MS literature that spoke to the considerable emotional distress that family members of someone with MS experienced[6-8] and encouraged him to attend group psychoeducation sessions for caregivers, which can prove beneficial.[9] In many ways, Bob had worked out some of this before he started coming to see me, but it helped to have his wife's doctor reiterate it because doing so validated his feelings and undercut his misplaced guilt. The sessions that seemed to help him the most were those devoted to the neurological explanations for Emma's dramatically altered behavior. It came as a revelation to him to learn that apathy was not willful stubbornness, a voluntary passive-aggressive response on his wife's part to her devastating illness, but rather a hardwired, uncontrollable character change brought about by damage to key anatomical regions and alterations in dopamine transmission, in particular.

Richard Marin has written extensively on the subject of apathy in general and devised a psychometric rating scale, the Apathy Evaluation Scale, that can be used by clinicians, informants, and individuals undertaking a self-assessment.[10] "Apathy," derived from the Greek adjective "apathēs," meaning without feeling, can arise as a *primary syndrome*, defined as a loss of motivation not attributable to emotional distress, intellectual impairment, or a diminished level of consciousness. A distinction is drawn between apathy as a syndrome and apathy as a *symptom*, also indicative of an amotivational state but in this case secondary to psychiatric or neurologic illness.[11,12] Apathy as a symptom can therefore be found in illnesses such as depression, Alzheimer's disease, and multiple sclerosis, to name but three. Neural connections associated with this behavioral change encompass the anterior cingulate, nucleus accumbens, ventrolateral globus pallidus, and the medial dorsal nucleus of the thalamus.[13] If the network is damaged, drive and motivation decline, and an indifference to life in general sets in.

"I don't give a damn about apathy," remarked Groucho Marx. This pithy and amusing word play is vintage Groucho, and while it cleverly encapsulates the subjective emotions, or rather lack thereof, experienced by the apathetic individual, Groucho Marx was clearly not referring to a profound degree of indifference that can characterize behavior in the context of a degenerative illness, like MS. For those who have to live with, and care for a person with MS-related apathy, there is nothing amusing at all about the condition. To the person with apathy, the very nature of the disorder means that the distress felt by their loved ones and friends is not personally experienced. Bob's emotional pain was on multiple levels: observing his wife's physical decline, witnessing her cognitive slide into dementia, and finally his sense of bemusement giving way to incredulity, hurt, and at times anger at her seeming indifference to it all and to how her illness was affecting her family.

The American Psychiatric Association (APA) has a diagnosis for this pathologic, all-embracing behavioral change in response to an acquired brain disease: namely, "personality change due to another medical condition."[14] Various subtypes of personality are listed, such as apathetic, aggressive, disinhibited, labile, and mixed, the last referring to more than one kind of behavioral disturbance. In Emma's case, the predominant feature was her disinterest in everything and everyone, including herself, which are the hallmarks of apathy. But every now and then, rousing herself from her blanket indifference, she would snap at Bob and their son in a most uncharacteristic display of anger, precipitated by something trivial or by nothing at all. And in those displays of pique, one saw elements of another personality subtype emerge with her verbal aggression.

Medical diagnoses can, paradoxically, give comfort. They provide an explanation, remove uncertainty, and validate what has, until then, been unfathomable. I use the word paradoxically here because even if the diagnosis is ominous, bringing with it a poor prognosis, for some people this is preferable to the limbo of uncertainty. A confirmed diagnosis comes with a rational explanation, and with it one is back on terra firma. Distressing as the diagnosis might be, planning for what the future holds can now begin with a greater certainty. Being diagnosed with a personality change secondary to her MS meant nothing to Emma. She lacked the insight to understand the consequences of the diagnosis, and her profound apathy left her indifferent to these consequences anyway. But to Bob, the diagnosis was little short of a revelation, even if the prognosis that came with it was grim. And grim it is, for there are few more intractable conditions in neuropsychiatry than a hardwired personality change arising in the context of a neurodegenerative disorder like MS. With the apathy superimposed on major cognitive decline, the best that Bob could hope for was a degree of palliation in an environment that was supportive, offered stimulation appropriate to Emma's reduced needs, and provided the requisite physical care and rehabilitation. The search was on for a nursing home, and hard as it was for Bob to say goodbye to the woman he had once known, he was able to begin the process unencumbered by worry, doubt, and anger that his wife's withdrawing from him and the occasional hard word directed at him were not signs of love disavowed, or disapproval of the care that he had labored to provide, but rather the consequences of a mind lost to illness and a personality altered beyond all recognition by it.

The APA approach to personality change is one way of describing the altered behavior that can come about in response to a disease like MS. There is, however, another way of defining personality attributes, one that is not rooted in pathological change as a consequence of illness. The five-factor model[15] holds that personality in general can be conceptualized as a combination of five basic traits: neuroticism, extraversion, conscientiousness, agreeableness, and openness to experience. Examples of each of these traits are as follows: neuroticism—anxious, tense; extraversion—talkative, outgoing, assertive; conscientiousness—organized, responsible, reliable; agreeableness—forgiving, generous, appreciative; and openness—curious, wide interests. To varying degrees, these traits are present in everyone. People with high extraversion and openness are typically outgoing, socially adept, and affable. They engage easily and with evident enjoyment in the world around them. They are well liked if they also scored high on the agreeableness scale. If not, the combination of high extraversion and low agreeableness could make the individual loud and bombastic and a person to dodge at social functions. And if this person is your boss, work could be an unpleasant place. But let us assume this particular individual is by nature open and agreeable as well. Take his developmental history and you will see that these character traits manifested early, during childhood, and were increasingly discernable by adolescence, when he would have been a popular kid in school who had many friends and even more acquaintances, and who was a favorite of his teachers.

Fast forward 30 years. Jim, our once gregarious young man, has well-advanced MS. He was given the diagnosis in his early 20s. The news upset him at first, but he soon bounced back, and his symptoms did not stop him from socializing actively. By his mid-20s, he was married to an equally outgoing woman, her vivaciousness in tune with his innate joie de vivre. The couple settled down to have a family, and they got on with their lives, learning to adapt to the relapses that came with the disease. Jim's physical decline was slow, but inexorable, with a cane giving way to a walker by the time he was referred to my clinic. By now, he was working from home, an accommodation provided by the same insurance company that had first employed him fresh out of university.

Jim's wife, Ellen, accompanies him to the appointment. She is the one who instigated the referral through their family doctor. Jim is nonplussed by this. When I ask him what the problem is, he shrugs, laughs uneasily, with his eyes revealing an absence of mirth, and begins telling me of his limb spasticity and the challenges that he now has with his walking. In the same breath, he wonders aloud how a psychiatrist can help him with this. As Jim talks, I observe him and Ellen closely. Jim is well groomed, neatly dressed, and still trim despite his sedentary life. His countenance is intermittently open and friendly, and his general demeanor offers glimpses of an earlier, boyhood charm. But overall, there is a wariness to his presentation that reflects his uncertainty about why he now finds himself in a psychiatrist's office. His eyes dart repeatedly to Ellen as he talks, betraying his unease, seeking out her reassurance.

Ellen sits beside Jim, eyes averted. She is surely aware of his discomfort but does nothing to allay it. She bides her time patiently until I have finished taking a history from him. Not once does she interrupt, confirm, or correct what he tells me. She, too, is well groomed and smartly dressed in a tailored suit, but unlike Jim, her expression shows no glimmer of lightness or hint of a smile, even if fleeting. Ellen's facial features are taught and her brow furrowed. Her bright red lipstick, immaculately applied, does nothing to soften the grim downturn to her mouth. The tension in their relationship is palpable. When it comes to Ellen's chance to talk, she is all business and cuts immediately to the chase. Without so much as acknowledging Jim's presence, she tells me they are not here to discuss his walking but rather his behavior. "This is not the man I married," she makes clear. With firm resolve and a vivisectionist's precision, she begins explaining why. Once upon a time, Jim had been outgoing, enjoyed people's company, and sought out new experiences. No longer. Once, he had shown ambition, taken on a challenge, overcome it, and moved on to the next one. Not anymore. To begin with, years back, early in their marriage, Jim had a romantic and loving side, one that made Ellen feel special, cared for, loved, and appreciated. This had all evaporated. For a moment, her resolve wavers and, on the verge of tears, she checks herself, dabs at the corner of her eyes with a tissue, and blows her nose before going on with her observations and a litany of complaints. Jim has become distant from their children. Their home has become a quiet, sad place. Friends seldom visit anymore because Jim just sits there, disengaged, and his indifference embarrasses them. This has forced Ellen to socialize on her own, away from home, and when in the company of other couples, she feels like a widow at times. She sees how their friends pity her, and she cannot stand it any longer. It is humiliating. She is still full of energy. Her work goes well. Life pulses all around her, and she wants to be part of it, to engage with it, to be caught up in the flow, and play her part, but instead it is all grinding to a halt, prematurely, as though old age has come calling 30 years too soon.

If these are tough accusations for Jim to hear, he shows no signs of it. Instead, he appears bemused and perplexed. What on earth is Ellen on about? As far as he is concerned, everything is fine except for his walking. If he could walk a little better, he could be more active and everything would be solved. Quick as a flash, Ellen has her riposte ready. This has nothing to do with walking. She is sympathetic to his difficulties here. She knows how hard it must be for him to schlepp around that collapsible walker of his. No, this has nothing to do with his ambulation. It is his attitude that is destroying their relationship. There is so much he could still do, walking aside. Travel, entertaining, movies, dining out, art appreciation classes—the list is endless and all of it possible within the confines of Jim's disability. But none of it is taking place. Their world has shrunk, life has slowed. A once vibrant and exuberant man has turned inward, disengaged from all but a few activities, working from home with accommodations, spending only a little time with the kids, a little TV, and early to bed. "It is crushing me," she confides softly. "My life is crushing me."

Ellen's history suggested a gradual transformation in Jim's personality over the past 20 years. But before I concluded as much, there were diagnostic pitfalls to avoid. Perhaps Jim's slow withdrawal from life indicated the presence of a disabling depression. So I asked a series of questions exploring this possibility, but drew a blank. Jim was steadfast in his denial of feeling sad, or despondent or miserable or any other kind of enduringly negative emotion. Sure, he admitted, his slow walking got him down from time to time, but his frustrations here were fleeting.

Having ruled out depression, I turned my attention to possible anxiety. Maybe this was the reason for his reluctance to engage in the types of activities Ellen has just described to me. Once more my inquiry came up empty. Sure, there were some things to worry about, but these concerns were fleeting. Anxiety had never been part of the clinical picture. It did not surface 20 years ago when Jim was first diagnosed, and it had not cropped up since.

The third diagnostic possibility to be considered was cognitive dysfunction. Perhaps this underlay Jim's inability to engage in activities previously enjoyed. At first glance, this seemed unlikely because Jim was still working full time, albeit from home. His accommodations appeared driven more by his problems with walking than anything else. It seemed unlikely that his company would show this degree of flexibility if he was not performing workwise. Still, a neuropsychological assessment was needed and duly completed. The results revealed some falloff in processing speed, considered mild. Visual memory was now impaired. Verbal memory and executive functions fell in the low normal range, a decline for a man with a high pre-MS intellect and robust cognitive reserve. The deficits, while wide-ranging, were for the most part mild and by themselves unlikely to account for Jim's character transformation.

With depression, anxiety, and marked cognitive dysfunction now ruled out as sole causative factors in Jim's behavioral change, what remained was a personality change. Jim's innate temperament had been altered by his MS. The extraversion that had been present when he was a young man was now seldom seen. Gone was his outgoing, gregarious nature, that spark which Ellen and a legion of friends had found so attractive. No longer was he open to new experiences, and his agreeableness, once the cornerstone of who he had been as a person, was slipping too. Jim was unaware of this. To him, it all boiled down to his walking. If he could ambulate freely like other people, everything would revert to how it had once been. But to Ellen, the change in Jim went way beyond his use of a cane or walker. She was right when, in her anguish, she had exclaimed, "This is not the man I married." Twenty years of inflammatory and degenerative changes in the brain had, bit by bit, transformed a once vibrant, socially adept, charming person. Outwardly, Jim still looked good. There was nothing in his appearance to indicate this transformation. His boyish handsomeness had not been lost. His weight had not ballooned with his sedentary lifestyle. He still showed flashes of his former self, in his smile, his occasional humorous aside, his insouciance in the face of adversity. But these markers of his former self were fleeting and misleading. There was no consistency to them. They had become the exception.

The process of change had been so slow to begin with—imperceptible at first, tiptoeing in by stealth—that it had been missed or else explained away euphemistically by Ellen and the family. "Jim is having a bad day" became the stock explanation for his lack of enthusiasm for an activity that he had once embraced with relish. As the years passed, the "bad days" became "bad weeks," and as life hurried on around him, Jim's engagement with it faltered. At first, his loved ones adapted to these changes. The social diary was rearranged. Holiday plans were altered but not canceled. Much of Ellen's attention focused on her young children in those hectic early years of starting a family, and Jim was content to follow, swept along in their wake. When he opted out of an engagement, he was missed, but nothing ominous was seen in his nonparticipation. After all, he had MS, and those two little letters carried all sorts of connotations about disability, never really discussed, but tacitly accepted as part of the new fabric of all their lives. Jim continued working, and going into the office gave his day structure and kept the rhythm of his life flowing, albeit slower now. His ability to work and bring in a good paycheck each month likely obscured some of the other subtler changes that were by now affecting his behavior, such as his less dominant role in conversations or his reduced drive when it came to going out on weekends or planning the family vacations. Previously, he had always taken the lead, searching out new adventures for them to explore.

As Jim slowly relinquished his assertive family role, Ellen picked up some of the slack, but not all of it. She was just too busy with her own career and raising the kids. Looking back now, she could see that her husband had been drifting from her and the family, but at the time she was not aware of it, distracted by the pace of her life and a to-do list that seemed endless. And then, one day, with her teenage children becoming increasingly independent and spending more time with friends than their mother, she was forced to take stock of her home situation. The dwindling dinner parties had ended some time back. Family vacations had stopped. Weekend outings were rare. Friends she had once considered close were now more distant. Her sexual life had withered, and Ellen could not recall when she and Jim had last been intimate. Loneliness was something new and a little frightening for her. At first, she reasoned that what had happened was typical for most families, that life takes over and rearranges one's priorities. But as she mulled this over, she could also see that her efforts at socializing and maintaining a family lifestyle that balanced work with play had been progressively spoiled by Jim. She hadn't pushed back when he had resisted and demurred. She had allowed him to set the pace of things, to dictate their recreational activities or lack of them. After all, she could see how his walking had slowed. And she had always admired his strength and resilience getting up each morning and pushing himself to go into the office, even when his legs seemed to be rebelling and he would rather have spent a little more time in bed because of his fatigue.

But she felt that now things had to change. Their finances were secure. The children were happy and doing well at school. Ellen and Jim were only in their mid-40s. There was a lot of time ahead that needed to be filled with good things. It was time to rebuild her relationship with her husband, become more active, put back a little spark, and rekindle what had once been a vibrant partnership. They would work around the challenges with his walking. She would take the lead. It was clear what needed to be done. They had a new game plan—well, it was hers really, but one that she felt sure he would embrace. After all, what was not to like in it? Filled with a new resolve, she sat Jim down and laid it all out. But he had no matching enthusiasm for anything she suggested. Indifference and reluctance greeted every new idea. From her perspective it was a response devoid of logic. Every one of her proposed initiatives was within his physical capabilities. None was welcomed. Shaken by Jim's response, Ellen recalled feeling angry at first, but this softened when she saw his confusion at her reaction. It was then that she became aware of having lost the man she had first fallen for. This newfound insight arrived like a hammer blow, but later that night, when alone with her thoughts, Ellen could see that it had been long in coming. She had avoided confronting it because the reality was simply too painful. Jim was no longer the person he had once been. It was as though his inner core had been shelled out, his dynamism, drive, and enthusiasm for life replaced by a hesitant, avoidant, and timid doppelganger. Two years on from this epiphany she finds herself in my office for the first time, and all the accumulated disappointments, frustrations, and hurt come spilling out.

If we apply the APA's diagnostic criteria for a personality change to Jim's presentation, we come up a little short. His lack of motivation, or apathy, is selective. He still takes good care of his appearance, works a full day, and brings in a good salary; he completes those housekeeping chores that have always been his responsibility and which he is still able to do, such as washing the dishes, mowing the lawn, even with his faltering gait, and putting gas in the car. Rather, the changes that have occurred relate to his reluctance to explore new things, an inability to engage on an emotional level, his indifference to social contacts, and a lack of curiosity—a stark contrast to his core pre-MS temperamental characteristics. While the apathy label would not be incorrect in describing aspects of Jim's behavior, the changes that have transformed his interpersonal relationships are more completely understood within the constructs of the five-factor personality approach.

Personality change in people with MS has not been well studied, but a small literature provides a consistent body of evidence that helps explain Jim's presentation. In a retrospective study of 67 people with MS, researchers found that educational and occupational achievement were associated with higher openness, whereas childhood social engagement was linked to extraversion, agreeableness, and conscientiousness.[16] Persistent evidence of extraversion was in turn associated with current involvement in exercise and social activities, whereas neuroticism correlated with engaging in hobbies. Here it is not hard to see Jim's developmental and clinical histories written large in these findings. The authors went on to report another significant observation—that childhood enrichment, a marker for cognitive reserve, and conscientiousness combined as predictors of cognitive processing speed after accounting for the effects of age, disease duration, level of physical disability, and the volume of cerebral gray matter.

The linkage between personality and cognition emerged once more in a study of 275 people with MS and 55 health controls which also used the NEO Five-Factor Inventory. A personality profile of higher neuroticism, lower extraversion, and lower conscientiousness was found in half the MS group but only 24% of the healthy sample.[17] These maladaptive personality changes, however, were only present in those people with MS who were also cognitively impaired. Another study that explored the relationship between cognition and personality in a sample of 80 people with MS reported that higher openness and lower neuroticism were associated with a better memory, even after controlling for the potentially confounding effects of age, brain atrophy, education, and IQ.[18] Lower conscientiousness, on the other hand, was linked to poorer memory.

There is also some tentative, indirect evidence that these personality characteristics are driven by structural brain changes induced by MS. In a study of 98 people with MS, Benedict et al.[19] showed that reduced gray matter volume and low conscientiousness were associated with cognitive impairment. They also, however, reported a novel finding; namely, that high neuroticism appeared to interact with gray matter atrophy in the development of euphoria, which in the MS literature refers to a fixed mental state characterized by a cheerful mood, optimistic outlook, and unrealistic sense of physical well-being, despite the presence of significant neurological disability.[20]

The four studies referenced here are cross-sectional, the assessments capturing a moment in time in which the elicited cognitive data were linked to current aspects of the person's personality. What remains unclear is whether the five-factor personality components identified are state or trait. Do they reflect the individual's core personality or have the structural and functional brain changes of multiple sclerosis brought about a shift in personality, amplifying or diminishing one or more factors? While the case histories of Emma and Jim provide strong anecdotal evidence of the disease eroding positive personality attributes, the only way to answer this question definitively is to undertake a longitudinal study, ideally over many years, because when personality changes in people with MS, it generally does so slowly, an accumulation of subtle shifts that at first may go unnoticed. Two studies have attempted this. In the first, the follow-up period was three years, and no longitudinal changes were recorded on the NEO Five-Factor Inventory.[21] However, when the study duration was extended to five years, evidence emerged of a decline in extraversion and conscientiousness, but only in those individuals whose cognition had also deteriorated over this period.[22]

More work is needed to tease out the relationship between personality on the one hand and disorders of cognition and behavior in people with MS on the other. This is a nascent area of MS research, as the attention of MS behavioral researchers over the past few decades has been focused elsewhere. Perhaps one reason for this lag may relate to the paucity of treatment options that are available to address the problem. There is no published treatment study of personality change secondary to MS. There appears to be a tacit understanding that by the time personality alters, the brain plasticity window has closed, leaving the behavioral changes irreversible. One can postulate that pharmacotherapy might soften the edges of neuroticism, energize the apathetic, or bring back a modicum of the agreeableness that has been lost, but to date there is no evidence to support this. Similarly, behavior modification techniques, while not put to the therapeutic test in an MS-related clinical trial, are likely to yield little given the potential fixity of the problem. Glimmers of hope may, however, be extracted from studies showing that cognitive behavior therapy in depressed people reduced neuroticism and increased extraversion,[23] while intensive mindfulness therapy for physicians to combat burnout led to increased conscientiousness and lower neuroticism.[24] Whether similar gains are possible in the context of the irreversible brain changes, in particular atrophy, associated with multiple sclerosis remains highly questionable.

The primary physician can feel helpless at times to alter the course of this behavioral decline. The fixity of the personality change coupled with a lack of insight and the progressive nature of the underlying disease means that interventions should be aimed at helping families come to terms with this bleak outcome. In my experience, the spouses of people like Emma and Jim often spare their children here, urging them to get on with their lives. But families are constituted differently. What happens when a spouse is deceased and the person with MS has gone to live with their child? Or what of the scenario where a partner has left—walked out on a 20-year relationship with the bitter parting words, "I never signed up for this!"—and a child is left to pick up the pieces? Now the onus of care falls elsewhere, and the strains that come with it are considerable.

I am witness to these quiet family sorrows playing out daily. And while the outcome in terms of symptom resolution is poor, there are other ways to measure how individuals respond to adversity. Bob never left Emma, even after she moved into the nursing home. He visited her every evening on his way to work. Ellen stayed with Jim too, painstakingly building a narrow, parallel life that left her time to be with him and share part of their evenings and weekends together. This is what I am witness to as well—the bonds of love and companionship that never break completely, even when the strains are great and aspects begin to fray. Time and again I see partners tap into their own deep wellsprings of resilience, learning as they go, adjusting the building blocks of day-to-day living to accommodate a new reality that circumstances have forced on them. It is deeply moving to observe this hesitant, painstaking journey toward acceptance, which begins with the realization that a partner has fundamentally, irrevocably changed. If this hurdle can be overcome, and it is here that the role of the therapist can prove crucial, then the relationship that emerges on the other side, while significantly altered, can provide not only companionship but some happiness too.

SEVEN

Sadness and Irritability

DEPRESSION IS A broad term. At one end of the spectrum, it refers to a symptom, as in, "I am feeling depressed." Here the word simply reflects the individual feeling of sadness, a universal human emotion that in the majority of people is transient and arises in response to hearing some upsetting news, witnessing a distressing event, or having a troubling thought. This fleeting emotion is not accompanied by the other symptoms that characterize a more ominous kind of sadness, one that falls at the other end of the spectrum. Here the sadness is pervasive and seldom lifts. Concomitant difficulties include an inability or reduced ability to enjoy life (also called anhedonia), changes in sleep (too little or too much) and appetite (either reduced or increased), negative thoughts about oneself or the future, guilt, low energy, and thoughts that life may not be worth living. When five or more of these symptoms accompany a persistently low mood for two weeks or more, then the diagnosis of major depression is made. This is a serious psychiatric illness that can have a negative impact of many aspects of a person's life, as we shall see. Between the two extremes of short-lived sadness, on the one hand, and pervasive, disabling depression, on the other, comes numerous gradations of low mood. Once more it is helpful to think of behavioral change, in this case depression, falling along a continuum.

Major depression is common in people with multiple sclerosis. Data collected from MS clinics suggest that the lifetime prevalence rate approaches 50%.[1-3] This means that one in two people with MS will develop a major depressive illness. More recent epidemiological findings confirm the high rates. The Canadian Community Health Survey[4] found a 12-month prevalence of 25.7% in people with MS whose ages fell in the 18–45 years range. This rate exceeded that found in people with other chronic illnesses. More recently, Marrie et al. surveyed 44,452 people with MS from four Canadian provinces and compared their psychiatric data to 220,849 individuals in the general population matched for age, sex, and geographical location.[5] The annual incidence of depression per 100,000 people was 979 in the MS group, 71% higher than that in the matched sample, when adjusted for year, sex, and age.

People with MS can experience a plethora of disabling symptoms affecting balance, strength, sensation, vision, bladder and bowel control, and sexual performance, not to mention cognition. Furthermore, there is no cure to MS. As one of my patients with MS trenchantly reminded me, you can say someone *had* cancer, but you can never say the same for MS. There is no past tense here. Once you get the disease, it will be with you in varying degrees of severity until the end of your life, which for someone with MS comes on average seven years earlier than in the general population.[6] MS is part of you, my patients tell me repeatedly, and their symptoms are a constant reminder of it. So, if you add the adjective "incurable" to a list of disabling symptoms, is it not understandable why depression arises so frequently? The answer here is both yes and no. Yes, because this reactive hypothesis does hold true for many people. No, because many people with MS will never become depressed. And to add another layer of complexity, some people with few if any physical symptoms will become profoundly depressed. This too should not be surprising. "Life is a complicated business, fraught with mystery and some sunshine," observed Philip Roth. To which a postscript could be added: "Welcome to the world of a person with MS."

What I plan to do in the following series of case reports is to illustrate the broad range of presentations that encompass depression in people with MS, shed some light on the mystery of why some people but not others succumb to depression, and then bring in the sunshine by showing how depression can, in some cases, be treated. Let me start with a common clinical presentation.

Lisa is 24 years old, single, working at a bank, and still living at home, saving her salary for a down payment on an apartment. She had always been healthy. After finishing high school, she soon found a bank job, her excellent people skills quickly apparent to prospective employers. She had started out as a teller but had aspirations to become a financial adviser, and she was in the process of completing course work and examinations to that end. Outside of work, she had a good circle of friends who would meet on weekends to party. Things were good at home. Both parents were well, and Lisa had a close relationship with them and her two younger siblings. In short, life was moving along smoothly, the five-year plan in place and attainable.

And then, one morning, Lisa wakes up blind in her right eye. The eye is painful too. She gets an appointment with her GP that afternoon; he is a kindly, gentle man, who has known her since she was a child. He takes one look into her eye and tells her to go the local emergency room. After a long wait, Lisa finally sees the neurology intern. It is close to midnight when she has her MRI. She finds the machine claustrophobic and has to fight a rising sense of panic as she lies there trying not to move as instructed. At three o'clock in the morning, in pain, half-blind, and dog-tired, Lisa is given the diagnosis of optic neuritis. "What does it mean?" she asks. "Well it's not MS yet," she is told, and she is given an appointment to see the neurologist that afternoon. By the time all the paperwork has been completed and a taxi found to take Lisa home, it is dawn. Her parents are waiting up anxiously for her. "What's the verdict, kid?" asks her dad, trying to sound chipper. "It's not MS yet," she repeats, on the verge of tears. Through her one good eye she sees the shock in her parents' faces. "What do you mean, not MS yet?" they chorus. Notwithstanding the long night, they all huddle around the computer while Lisa's father searches "optic neuritis." Lisa finds it painful to look at the screen because of the bright light. In silence, the family scrolls through a number of websites. By the time Lisa falls asleep—the pain in her eye numbed by a hefty dose of paracetamol—she has learned one thing about her lost vision: it is the presenting symptom of multiple sclerosis in 20% of cases.[7] One in five. She wonders if that is good or bad.

Lisa wakes up at midday, feeling exhausted and still blind in the one eye, which remains painful. Mom has stayed home from work to go with her to the neurologist. The appointment goes well. The neurologist does not hurry. His manner is calm, gentle, and reassuring. He repeats the neurological examination familiar to Lisa from the night before and tells her that, apart from her visual changes, everything else is fine. She is told she does not have MS but is at risk of developing the disorder now that she has optic neuritis. Her mother intervenes wanting a more definite answer. None is forthcoming. It is their first introduction to a new world of uncertainty, one that in time becomes familiar to people with MS. When will my next attack occur? When will my symptoms get worse? Or improve? Do these symptoms end in a wheelchair? So many questions met by answers always couched in probabilities and statistics.

There is, however, no equivocation when it comes to treating her optic neuritis. A short course of intravenous steroids is recommended. She can start today. And so it is that she soon finds herself sitting in a plastic armchair with a needle in her arm as fluid drips slowly into her vein. She arranges to take a two-week leave of absence from work. Social events are canceled. Apologies are texted to colleagues on her volleyball team—she cannot make this evening's match. A little more than 24 hours have passed since she awoke partially blind. How can it be, she asks herself, that I can go to bed one evening in robust health and wake up to this nightmare? Life has turned on a dime, and she feels herself floundering.

Four days later, things start looking up. The course of steroid is finished, the pain is gone, and about 80% of her vision has returned to her right eye. This rapid improvement lifts Lisa's spirits. Family and friends have rallied around, and for the first time in days she can shift her thinking away from her health. When the time comes to return to work, her colleagues greet her warmly. She has been missed.

Lisa picks up where she left off, but things are not quite the same. To begin with, her vision is still a little fuzzy. Will it ever come back? Her neurologist cannot say for sure. She also feels a little fatigued, which is a new sensation, because she has always been a high-energy person. When midafternoon arrives, she would give anything for a short nap. A double espresso is now her drug of choice, she jokes. There is also that niggle of anxiety about another attack. But as the days run into weeks and then months, her health holds firm. Work goes well, and she passes her next-to-last exam with an excellent grade. She is back on the volleyball team, and Saturday nights are seldom spent at home. Even her fatigue is starting to fade, pushed aside by a lifestyle that is quickening in step with her ambitions.

When the numbness in her leg starts, it is so subtle at first she doesn't make the connection with her earlier episode of lost vision. Perhaps it was because the sensation was not new. She had had brief episodes like this over the years, and they had always resolved quickly. This time it is different. The numbness worsens, and she takes to pinching herself hard to elicit any feeling in the region. Within a week the diagnosis of MS is confirmed.

Lisa recalls the moment she was given her diagnosis. She knew it was coming. Time on the internet had spelled out the diagnostic criteria days before she saw her neurologist. Being armed with this certainty does not, however, soften the blow of confirmation. To her surprise, when she gets the news she bursts into tears. Much of the visit is spent sobbing, she recalls, so that by the time she leaves the office, she has been given not only a prescription for a disease-modifying drug but an appointment to see me too.

She enters my office with a bright, tense smile. It is a mask I have seen countless times before in people coming to their first psychiatric consultation. Beneath the bright, well-groomed exteriors are seas of emotions held in check by many factors: willpower, pride, fear of appearing weak, perhaps distrust? Whatever the reasons, time will reveal them, as it will the emotions that compete with this resolve. Over the course of the next hour with Lisa, a familiar theme with variations unfolds. A young life has been upended by disease. And because multiple sclerosis is so common in Canada, almost everyone knows a person with it, be it a relative, a friend, or the mother of a friend. If that person is disabled, which is often the case, then it is the image of a walker or a wheelchair that looms large over this first consultation.

There is often, however, some good news to be imparted at this point. The symptoms of depression may be transient, wedded to the sudden uncertainty over what the future now holds. Lisa's low mood is distractible. Friends come around to visit and spirits pick up. The family goes on an outing and her mood lightens. Sleep may be fragmented, but appetite is unchanged, and the beliefs that are typically linked to a major depression, such as guilt and poor self-esteem, are absent. Lisa, like so many people newly diagnosed with an incurable, potentially disabling condition, is understandably frightened by the unexpected turn her life has taken.

There is one more variation to the theme that needs highlighting. Six months back, Lisa had not a care in the world. Overnight, optic neuritis rendered her blind in one eye. She bounced back from this, albeit incompletely, but just as she is finding her footing and righting her life, a leg goes numb and she is diagnosed with MS. Two big stressors back-to-back, and a new concern has been added. She has been referred to a psychiatrist. "Does this mean I have become mentally unwell too?" she wonders. I often come across this worry at a first consultation. The fear of mental instability compounding the fear of multiple sclerosis. There it lies, this composite worry, just beneath the bright smile that soon cracks, smudging her cheeks with mascara-tinged rivulets.

There is much to be accomplished at this first appointment. Obtain a detailed history, complete the mental state examination, arrive at a diagnosis if possible, and then, in the time remaining, reassure Lisa that what she is experiencing emotionally is common to people with newly diagnosed MS. Feeling upset and worried—and yes, depressed for short periods—is a natural reaction to adverse news of this consequence. In the absence of a formal psychiatric illness, it is important not to

pathologize what she is feeling. At the same time, it is incumbent to offer support and guidance, if needed, in developing the coping strategies
that she will require for a lifetime. Here, the therapist is on firmer ground
empirically, for there is persuasive research as to which kinds of coping
strategies work and which are harmful. But more of that later. As for
Lisa, her distress settled in the weeks that followed. She only needed
a few sessions of supportive therapy, from which she emerged with a
new rallying cry. Carpe diem. Seize the day. She also began her disease-
modifying medication, eased back into work with a graduated return,
and picked up her socializing. Lisa never shed her neurological diagnosis of course, but her disease was in remission and life, for the moment
at least, was being led to the full.

The evolution and speedy resolution of Lisa's depression is a familiar clinical history, common to many people with MS. Seldom does a
clinic goes by in which I do not come across a person with MS whose
depression is triggered by the sudden onset of a disabling symptom that
came out of nowhere, without warning or prodrome, forever altering a
life in which one of the few certainties now is uncertainty. The precipi-
tous arrival of blindness or paralysis or incapacitating dizziness in a
healthy 30-year-old person can easily overturn assumptions about health
and call into question future plans by revealing, decades too soon, that
life is indeed fragile and one's mortality uncomfortably close. No surprise, then, that depression can quickly follow, for uncertainty and vulnerability offer a rich breeding ground. However, as Lisa showed so
clearly, resilience may be marginally slower out the gates but, when present, overrides worry and sadness with advantageous coping strategies
that are either innate or learned through therapy.

What happens, however, when resilience falters in the face of physical
disability? When coping strategies are dysfunctional and the shadow of
disease blots out the sunshine?

Roza is in hear early 50s, married with two grown daughters who
live independently. Her husband is a successful businessman and there
are no financial worries. She has had MS for 10 years, and it has entered a secondary progressive phase. Her biggest difficulty is spasticity,

which has hobbled her walking. Movement is now very difficult, each step effortful and painfully slow. She has been referred to me for her depression.

I find her sitting outside my office before her first appointment. She is well dressed and coiffed, and my first impression is of an elegant woman. She rises unsteadily from her seat and fumbles awkwardly for an elaborately painted cane that has slipped to the floor. She almost falls in the process. I move to help her, but with her one free hand she brusquely waves me away. Stepping back, I wait for her to enter my office. It is a laborious process. First, the right leg shuffles spasmodically forward, where it stops to await the cane, which soon arrives. With the cane in place as anchor, the left leg begins its arduous journey inching forward, accompanied by a scuffing sound as her shoe scrapes along the carpet. Now with her two limbs aligned and the cane wedged in place, the process repeats itself, the right leg jerking loose, the cane following, the left leg—which remains stationary until called on—to follow. All the while, Roza's body is bent over at a 45-degree angle, but she holds her head high, a look of fierce, grim determination in her eyes.

It is perhaps no more than eight steps from the door of my office to a comfortable chair. It is a journey that takes a more mobile person a couple of seconds. Unthinking seconds. An action that is taken for granted, so simple, repeated countless times in different situations. We enter room, saunter over to a chair, sit down, make ourselves comfortable. Who stops to think about it, analyze what we have just done, break it down into segments that need to be planned and navigated? Actions such as these, automatic, unconscious, essentially effortless, keep us moving from object to object, place to place. We never give them a second thought. Not only do we have the blessing of unfettered movement, we can also instantly, instinctually modify our speed. On a leisurely day we amble. To catch the bus when late for work, we run. To keep up with an energetic friend, we increase the pace of our stride. Infinite gradations of speed, achieved without a thought, adjusted spontaneously to the task at hand. And there is so much more to marvel at, if we are forced to stop and think about it, as Roza has to. We are constantly fine-tuning our movements, and that of course includes our walking. We skip over the crack in a sidewalk, step aside adroitly to avoid getting splashed by a passing car on a rainy day, shift to either side in a busy pedestrian thoroughfare. Actions like these, repeated countless times, slow when we climb into bed at night and rest from a ceaseless variety of movements we have never thought about. And even then, tucked in under the sheets and in repose, movement does not stop. We need to get comfortable, legs shift, weight is redistributed, even on the most comfortable of mattresses. Or an itch has started up on an ankle and must be scratched, and to reach it, the leg must be bent and brought closer to the hand, and as we all know, an itch can be difficult to ignore. We move less at night, but we never stop moving for long, and who ever gives these nocturnal limb meanderings much thought?

Then one day a wrench is thrown in the works of our supremely efficient motor system. On a frigid winter's day, you step off a sidewalk onto some black ice, turn your ankle, and fall. Nothing is broken, thankfully, and there is no neurological damage, but the ligament sprain is so painful it is difficult to walk. You must wear a walking boot to support the bruised soft tissue, and the cheery orthopedic surgeon advises you to keep it on for at least six weeks. You limp away from the doctor's office in the clunky boot, cane in hand to ease the weight on the foot, and suddenly life is very different. You are hobbled. You have to be careful every time you place your foot on the ground because if you relax your vigilance a shard of pain shoots up your limb and makes you wince. Getting in and out a car is a real bother with the cumbersome boot. A shower is taken sitting down. You only move in first gear now and so consciously have to budget more time for everything. This means getting up half an hour earlier to get to work on time. If late, you will now miss the bus. On a rainy day, you are the one who is more likely to get splashed and have a soggy trouser leg. At a friend's party you cannot join the revelry on the dance floor and instead watch from the sidelines, where from time to time, someone throws you a bone of commiseration before wheeling away to rumba some more. So many small inconveniences, irritations, newfound obstacles to overcome. What makes it all bearable, of course, is the knowledge that it is time-limited, that in a few weeks the boot will be gone, and with a little physiotherapy you will again be able to sprint for the morning bus, bound up the stairs before the driver closes the doors behind you, slip your token into the slot, and without a second thought make your way down the swaying, lurching aisle to a free seat in the far back corner, which you reach by dexterously stepping over a bulging backpack. It is all so easy, not worth a second thought, the twisted ankle no more than a distant memory, a blip in time. Life is back on track, and movement is once again fast, coordinated, efficient, and effortless. We just don't think about it because the whole physical apparatus, driven by an intact nervous system unencumbered by muscle weakness, is in good order. Our thoughts are elsewhere, given freedom to revert to higher-order cognitive tasks, like problem solving at work, abstractions, or organizing activities. The basic building blocks of movement are taken for granted, allowing us the freedom to put into effect the actions our intellects demand.

But not for Roza. No transient disability here. Her problem is not primarily muscular or ligamentous; it is neurological. Not only will there be no recovery, further deterioration is likely. There is nothing automatic or effortless about her movement now, and it has been this way for years. Every step is an effort, calling on a conscious resolve to keep moving, placing one obstinate, disobedient leg in front of the other, pushing through the stiffness and pain that ambulation now entails. All the myriad spin-offs that come with free and easy movement have been lost. And she is reminded of this every time she needs to take a step. In the therapy sessions that followed, I would come to appreciate that this unceasing challenge, from which she has no respite, had come to define her existence. An early hint of the therapeutic challenge that lay ahead, however, could be gleaned from her facial expression on the morning of our first meeting as she dragged herself over to the chair. A mishmash of anger, resolve, and defiance, which never wavered.

As I got to know Roza better, it became clear to me that her illness was all consuming. If one looked beyond the MS, there were so many good aspects to her life. A loving and supportive husband, a beautiful home adapted to her physical limitations, financial security, and a rehabilitation worker on hand when needed. The luxurious circumstances of her adult life were a continuation of a charmed childhood. Born into wealth and a loving family, Roza had sailed through school with good grades, lots of friends, and numerous awards, both academic and athletic. Vacations had always been fun—in the summer, at a family cottage on a pristine, secluded lake, or in the winter, in the mountains of Whistler, British Columbia, where her parents kept what was euphemistically referred to as a ski cabin. There was never any shortage of boyfriends, and her choice, made when she was 21 years of age, fell on a young man whose circumstances and upbringing were essentially a carbon copy of her own. Two families blessed with wealth, good looks, strong bonds, and robust health coming together. No wonder the inlaws on both sides were so delighted with the match.

More good fortune followed. Two healthy children were born, and after spending a few years at home with them until they were settled in school, Roza opened her own business designing high-end leather goods. The company flourished with the goods manufactured in Mexico and sold worldwide through online shopping and flagship stores in the Toronto, New York, and Milan. It was while visiting her factory in Chiapas that Roza first became aware of something wrong with her gait. One of her legs was a little weak. She brushed it off to begin with, but later that year, while celebrating her 41st birthday with a small gathering of friends at a favorite restaurant she stumbled and fell on some stairs. The weakness could no longer be ignored. It took another year for the diagnosis of MS to be confirmed. She recalls feeling stunned when she got the news. MS? Surely not. There was no place for news like this in her life—41 years of unsullied health and good fortune so rudely interrupted. She remembers refusing to accept the diagnosis. A second opinion was quickly sought at the Mayo Clinic, where MS was just as quickly confirmed. "Well," she remembers thinking, "a disease might have laid claim to me, but I will fight it by ignoring it." Shock had given way to anger and defiance.

No sooner is the diagnosis made than coping mechanisms begin. For many people, stunned by the diagnosis, these first coping steps are instinctive as they draw on innate strategies that they have used over the course of their lives until now. Given that MS generally begins in young or middle-aged adults, the news of having the disease will be for many people the biggest medical challenge confronted so far. How they cope with the disease and adapt to it has the potential to define a large part of their lives and, by extension, those of their partners, parents, and children as well. Not surprisingly, coping skills are closely linked to depression and anxiety and emotional wellness.

There is a large literature devoted to coping with multiple sclerosis. Broadly speaking, coping strategies can be adaptive or maladaptive. Within this division are to be found specific approaches that break down into three broad categories: problem-focused, emotion-focused, and avoidant-focused strategies. Their nomenclature will vary according to the psychometric scales used to detect them. For example, the Ways of Coping Index refers to planful problem solving, cognitive reframing, emotional respite, and escape avoidance. While the data associating depression with particular coping strategies are not unequivocal, there is a broad degree of agreement that problem-focused adaptation is good from a mental health perspective, whereas avoidance is not. The data for emotion-focused coping are more mixed.

The benefits of a problem-solving coping style were shown in a study of 101 people with MS with varying degrees of physical disability.[8] The greater the disability, the higher the depression scores. Avoidant and emotion-based coping were also associated with more depression, whereas planful problem solving was linked to lower levels of depression. Of note was that the relationship between less depression and focused problem solving was strongest in those people with the most advanced disability. Another interesting observation was the association between cognitive reframing, which reflects the attempts by an individual to acquire a new perspective on a problem, and lower depression scores. Other researchers have also found a relationship between the type of coping strategy used and the degree of neurological disability, with adaptive coping most prominent in individuals with Expanded Disability Status Scale (EDSS) scores between 3.0 and 6.0 indicative of moderate impairments.[9] This finding, unrelated to depression, was interpreted as evidence of individuals focusing more intensely on their challenges as their disability progressively increased. A different result, however, was reported by Lorefice et al.,[10] who found that as EDSS levels increased, avoidance linked to a past diagnosis of depression became more prominent. An analogous conclusion was noted by Arnett et al.,[11] who found that elevated rates of depression in cognitively impaired people with MS were accompanied by coping strategies high on avoidance and low on active coping interventions.

The harmful consequences of avoidant coping can be seen in unemployment data. A Norwegian study of 108 people with MS who were followed for 13 years showed that avoidance significantly and independently reduced the time to unemployment.[12] This finding is supported by a study showing that people with MS who resorted to behavioral disengagement, a coping style defined by a tendency to reduce effort or give in when confronted by a problem, were more likely to consider leaving work or to request reduced hours at work.[13] Allied to behavioral disengagement is a personality structure that contains higher neuroticism and lower extraversion.[13] These results, unrelated to depression, do not negate the much-replicated bidirectional association of low mood and unemployment that is present in the general psychiatry literature.[14,15]

While there is considerable supporting evidence for the benefits of problem-focused coping on depression,[16–19] a more tailored approach may be required in relation to certain stressors. In particular, when people with MS were confronted with uncontrollable stress, problem-focused strategies proved ineffective.[20] Instead, symptoms of depression and anxiety decreased when a meaning-focused approach was adopted. This is considered emotion-oriented, as it entails efforts to cope with difficult emotions by promoting acceptance and finding meaning within challenging life events. What this result also reveals is that the label "emotion-based" is broad, encompassing strategies that are both helpful, like the example given above, and unhelpful, like persistently venting one's emotions. This grab bag of approaches collated under one broad descriptor may explain, in part, the equivocal findings relating to emotion-focused coping in the MS behavioral literature. Less equivocation is present, however, with avoidant-focused coping, which is generally[16,21,22] but not always[23] considered unhelpful.

The MS coping literature, informative as it is, must be interpreted alongside a host of variables that can also modify how well people with MS adapt to their disease. These include external factors, such as finances, relationships, housing, leisure pursuits, the urban-rural health care divide, and personal characteristics like self-efficacy and resilience. Self-efficacy was defined by Bandura[24] and refers to a person's belief in his or her ability to carry out behaviors that are required to reach specific goals. As such, it is indicative of an individual's confidence in being able to exert a degree of control over his or her behavior and social milieu. The importance of this concept in adapting to a disabling disease like MS is reflected by the availability of at least four validated MS-specific self-efficacy scales.[25-28] There is evidence connecting greater self-efficacy with self-report metrics like reduced loneliness, a better quality of life, and improved physical, cognitive, and social functioning. The association with depression, however, is more equivocal,[29-33] reflecting a complex pathogenesis and methodological failings rather than conceptual shortcomings.

Resilience refers to the process of adapting well in the face of adversity. The latter can take many forms for a person with MS, as the case histories reveal thus far. The resiliency literature pertaining to the general vicissitudes of life is extensive, but it is much smaller for people with multiple sclerosis. In a longitudinal study, 163 people with MS were assessed at four points over the course of one year.[34] The data collected at each time point included indices of resiliency, social support (from significant others, family, and friends), depression, anxiety, and perceived general mental health status. While social support in its various forms was significantly associated with numerous aspects of mental wellness, the gist of the findings was that this relationship was almost entirely mediated by resilience. The study's longitudinal design gives these conclusions added weight and sheds welcome light on a substantial social-support depression literature in people with MS that is cross-sectional, and from which causal assumptions therefore cannot be inferred. The relative paucity of research devoted to resilience in people with MS and the importance of the concept makes this a fertile area for further research. One recent, welcome development has been the publication of the Multiple Sclerosis Resiliency Scale, the first of its kind for people with MS.[35]

Now that we are better acquainted with coping strategies used by people facing adversity, let us return to Roza and her struggles with multiple sclerosis. We can see that her inability to shift from an avoidant coping strategy was stoking her depression. This rigidity was not the product of impaired cognition, as neuropsychological testing had revealed mild, circumscribed deficits. Sadness now clouded much of her day. Her enjoyment of life was muted, and her self-esteem faltered in tandem with her labored gait. Sleep, too, had become problematic with early morning waking. Those first few hours of the day were the worst, she told me. She now had her own bedroom, for she could no longer bear her husband's uxorious solicitations. "His kindness was killing me," she complained. "It's a constant reminder of my limitations and frailties." So she moved into the guest suite, silently dismissing his concerns. When she awoke now, habitually around 4 a.m., she was alone. It was dark and the house was still. No sooner was she aware of her surroundings than a great sadness washed over her, accompanied by a feeling of tension and dread. How was she to face the day? If only she could stay in bed all day. There was nothing to look forward to. Her business had been handed over to someone else to manage. A temporary measure, she was told, when it became clear she was not up to the fast-paced job. Well, losing control of the business was the least of her problems, she reasoned. Soon the night would end and with daybreak came her first great challenge: limbering up and getting her legs moving enough to swing them over the side of the bed as a prelude to sitting. The stiffness was unbearable, always worse after a night lying down. There followed the shuffle to the bathroom—accomplished without cane, for she was determined to get to her first pee of the day without any assistive devices. "A pee on my terms alone," she told me defiantly.

The first few therapy sessions passed with little progress. Roza refused to take antidepressant medication. "It won't help me walk, and I am sad because I can't walk, so what's the use?" she asked, irritably. The talk therapy ran into the same immovable defiance. And yet, she kept coming to her appointments, always on time, meticulously groomed, and for much of the time spent with me, she railed against life, her fury interspersed with moments of tearfulness. It soon became apparent that my office was the only "safe place" where she allowed herself to express her grief. Each session became a cathartic outpouring of that week's stored up frustrations and emotional pain. No sooner was the time up than the mask was replaced and the barriers restored. "Just give me a minute," she would ask, as I brought the session to a close. She dabbed at her eyes, whipped out the vanity mirror and powder compact, expertly tidied her makeup, and voila, she was ready to face the world again, game face back on.

Two months into therapy, Roza's armor cracked, and she asked about medication for her depression. With this breakthrough, the conversation turned to a discussion of the various antidepressant agents and the best option for her. She had many questions, but the literature was found wanting when it came to answers. Despite clinically significant depression being so common in people with MS, there is a small evidence-based literature on antidepressant use in this disease. A Cochrane Review lists just three studies that meet the methodological bar for inclusion.[36] The first of these involved a tricyclic drug, a medication that dates back to the 1950s. In a randomized controlled study, Schiffer and Wineman[37] assigned 14 people with MS to a five-week trial of desipramine and individual psychotherapy and another 14 people to placebo and psychotherapy. Improvements in the desipramine group were found on the Hamilton Rating Scale for Depression but not on the Beck Depression Inventory. Difficulties tolerating side effects, such as dry mouth, constipation, and postural hypotension, were noted and prevented half the treatment group reaching what was considered a therapeutic dosage.

The second study that made it into the Cochrane Review involved the selective serotonin reuptake inhibitor (SSRI) paroxetine.[38] In a double-blind placebo-controlled trial, 42 people with MS and a confirmed diagnosis of major depression were randomly assigned to one of two parallel treatment groups—that is, paroxetine or placebo. Paroxetine was started at a dose of 10 mg once a day and titrated up to 40 mg per day depending on clinical response over the course of the

12-week intervention. Both groups improved with treatment. Thus, 57.1% of the paroxetine group and 40% of the control group had at least a 50% reduction in scores on the Hamilton Rating Scale for Depression, the study's primary outcome marker, a difference that did not reach statistical significance, probably due the small sample size. Side effects from the medication were again frequent and included nausea, headache, dry mouth, and sexual difficulties.

The third study included in the Cochrane Review compared another SSRI, sertraline, to two forms of psychotherapy—cognitive behavior therapy and supportive-expressive therapy[39]—and will be discussed later in this chapter. In addition to these three randomized controlled trials, there is a larger literature of open label and anecdotal reports attesting to the effectiveness of antidepressant medications across drug classes, including SSRI drugs (fluoxetine,[40,41] citalopram,[41] and sertraline[42]), a selective noradrenergic reuptake inhibitor (SNRI) medication (venlafaxine[41]), and a monoamine oxidase inhibitor (moclobemide[43]). Side effects can limit dosing. Particularly troubling are sexual difficulties, which are common in people with MS to begin with, affecting between 54% and 80% of individuals.[44,45] It is not uncommon for me to hear from a person with MS reporting an improvement in mood on an SSRI only to complain of newly acquired impotence.

There is a wide choice of antidepressant medications available, but in the absence of comparative studies, there are no data attesting to the benefits of one over another. What is known, however, is that these drugs have different therapeutic and pharmacokinetic profiles that can help steer the prescriber in a certain direction.[46] For example, if depression is linked to neuropathic pain, duloxetine and venlafaxine should be considered. If insomnia and nausea are considerations, mirtazapine would be a good choice. Bupropion and mirtazapine are drugs of choice if sexual difficulties are a concern. Should compliance with treatment be an issue, fluoxetine with its longer half-life will ensure that a missed dose here or there has less clinical significance. In the presence of cognitive difficulties, vortioxetine is an option. While there are no MS-related data on the drug, findings from an eight-week, double-blind, randomized, fixed-dose, placebo-controlled trial in a sample of 602 depressed adults demonstrated significant cognitive gains across multiple domains, including speed of processing, executive function, and memory.[47] A random effects meta-analysis has confirmed the cognitive benefits of vortioxetine relative to placebo and another antidepressant drug, duloxetine.[48]

I laid out the various antidepressant options to Roza, and we whittled the choice down to either mirtazapine, given her poor sleep, or duloxetine, because of the discomfort that came with her spasticity. In the end she went with mirtazapine. It certainly helped with her insomnia, and her crying stopped, but her mood never budged. If this seems contradictory given the absence of tears, it is not, for here one makes a distinction between mood (what a person feels subjectively) and affect (the outward display of emotion witnessed by others). The two are not always congruent, as we will see in Chapter 9. Antidepressant medication may therefore blunt a person's affect, preventing crying but without necessarily lifting sadness. This is what happened with Roza. The core features of her depression remained, as they did when the mirtazapine was switched to duloxetine after a failed two-month trial at therapeutic doses.

I had hoped that medication, if not completely alleviating Roza's depression, would at least allow her to begin addressing her disability and the many limitations that came with her labored gait. This was not to be. Her inability to walk freely was seen as a curse, undeserved and unfair. Rather than plan how to counteract her limitations and work around them, she chose to avoid the subject altogether. Avoidance in turn shrunk her world. Gone were the theater, movies, restaurants, dinner parties, and social functions. Her rationale for removing herself from society in this manner was to prevent people pitying her. How she hated the way strangers stared at her as she dragged around her insubordinate legs. She saw the looks on their faces, a mix of shock, surprise, sympathy, and morbid fascination. It was humiliating.

With medication having failed, I suggested she start seeing a colleague of mine who specialized in cognitive behavior therapy, or CBT. First developed by Aaron Beck in Philadelphia in the early 1960s, CBT is based on the premise that depressed people think in a certain "depressed" way. Thoughts can be distorted by low mood and a number of assumptions made that are false and that perpetuate the sadness. The aim of therapy is to identify these cognitive distortions, or negative beliefs, and correct them. This in turn can have a beneficial effect on mood. It is a practical therapy geared toward helping people with depression develop insights into their way of thinking and providing them with the tools to modify their negative thoughts. The skills learned during therapy can then be applied, not only to the depression currently experienced but also to any future episodes of depression that might arise, for depression is known to run a recurring course.

There is now a substantial body of evidence supporting CBT as an effective treatment for depression in people with MS. In an influential, early study by Mohr et al., 63 people with MS were randomly assigned to one of three treatment groups: CBT, supportive-expressive group therapy, or medication with the SSRI antidepressant drug sertraline.[39] The dosage of the sertraline was adjusted individually for maximum benefit (daily dosage range of 25–200 mg). After 16 weeks of therapy, the results showed that CBT and sertraline were equally effective and better than supportive-expressive therapy in reducing the number of people with major depression and lowering scores in some of the self-report psychometric mood scales. The dropout rates across the three treatment groups were 5%, 18%, and 29%, respectively, considered clinically significant but falling short of statistical significance because of the small sample size. Most telling, when participants were assessed six months after completing therapy, the benefits of CBT and sertraline were maintained.

A year before these data were published, Mohr et al.[49] had shown that CBT could be given effectively over the telephone in a study involving 32 depressed people with MS. Individuals receiving CBT showed a significant drop in mood-related symptoms compared to those in the usual-care control group. An added benefit that accrued from treatment was an improved adherence rate for the disease-modifying drug interferon beta-1α. The success of this eight-week intervention led to a more substantial study confirming the benefits of telephone-administered CBT.[50] The improved methodology included 16 weeks of treatment, a much larger sample size of 127 participants with MS, and a control group that was given supportive emotion-focused therapy rather than usual care, the latter often synonymous with no treatment at all. CBT once again outperformed supportive therapy across numerous outcome metrics, such as fewer people with major depression and lower scores in self-report measures of mood. Benefits were still present 12 months after completing therapy, although by then, between-group differences were no longer apparent.

Over the past 20 years, researchers have replicated David Mohr's important studies, showing that CBT for people with MS can be administered effectively to individuals[51,52] and in a group setting.[53,54] In addition, there are now computerized CBT programs for self-administration, four of which (Deprexis, MoodGYM, Beating the Blues, and MS Invigor8) have been trialed to promising effect in people with MS.[55] And the benefits may not stop here. While CBT was first developed by Aaron Beck with the aim of treating depression, there is evidence the core principles may be helpful to people with MS who have insomnia,[56] chronic pain,[57,58] and fatigue.[59]

More than 60 years have elapsed since Beck first formulated the principles of CBT. Over time, various offshoots have developed, one of which entails behavioral activation. In this intervention, the therapeutic emphasis shifts from changing the distorted thought patterns that influence mood to altering behaviors that affect mood. Evidence from the general psychiatry literature attests to the benefits of this simplified approach, with behavioral activation proving just as effective and a lot cheaper than CBT in treating individuals with major depression.[60] Preliminary data suggest that this approach may also help people with MS who are depressed.[61]

Another psychological therapy, mindfulness-based intervention, may also prove helpful in depression. The principle behind mindfulness therapy is to help individuals focus their attention on the present-moment experience. One hears echoes of Churchill's sage advice to command the moment to remain. In doing so, individuals can become more aware of thoughts, feelings, and actions that can hinder their progress through life. There are two specific types of mindfulness interventions: mindfulness-based stress reduction[62] and mindfulness-based cognitive therapy.[63] A recent systematic review pertaining to mental well-being (depression, anxiety, and stress) in people with MS identified 12 randomized controlled studies of sufficient quality to be included in the analysis.[64] As with CBT, the mindfulness interventions had been given individually, in group settings, in person, and online for periods that were generally briefer than for CBT, ranging from six to nine weeks. Effect sizes (they tell us the degree to which two groups differ) were moderate when compared to inactive placebo interventions and weak, but still positive, when the comparators were active.

There is a consistency to the CBT, mindfulness-based interventions, and antidepressant findings. They all help, albeit modestly. The American Academy of Neurology takes a more stringent view of the data, concluding that there is only weak evidence for one intervention, telephone-administered CBT.[65] A more recent systematic review and meta-analysis, however, paints a rosier picture, citing positive data from three drug and nine psychotherapy studies.[66] There are also other ways of looking at these positive findings. Stressful life events may lead to an exacerbation in MS,[67] so any intervention that helps an individual better manage stress may come with additional benefits beyond those conferred on mood. Furthermore, in a powerful affirmation of the mind-body connection, psychological interventions in people with MS have been shown to influence physical symptoms, most notably insomnia, pain, fatigue, and a sense of vitality.[68] Finally, data from another disabling disease have shown how mindfulness interventions, in particular, can reduce depression and anxiety and boost quality of life in caregivers to people with amyotrophic lateral sclerosis.[69]

I would like to report that 16 weeks of CBT with a skilled therapist shifted Roza's entrenched and maladaptive beliefs about her MS, but it did not. She returned to see me with that same grim, fierce resolve unchanged. She was at war with her disease, but it was not a battle she could win. Her inability to command the moment to remain, to look her tenacious adversary squarely in the eye and plan how to reduce its functional impact, meant she was in constant retreat. When she discontinued her antidepressant, the tears returned. At that point she stopped coming to see me. I offered to make a referral to another therapist, recognizing that even if her thinking was resistant to change, having a weekly opportunity to talk about her disease in a way she could not with those close to her might offer some comfort. She rejected this too. Avoidance had constricted her world to the confines of her home and a dwindling circle of immediate family and a couple of childhood friends who simply refused to be rebuffed.

As noted earlier, the diagnosis of major depression requires the presence of at least five symptoms for a minimum of two weeks. What is one to make of a clinical scenario in which the threshold is not met and only three of four symptoms are present? This clinical situation, referred to as subsyndromal depression, is common in psychiatry and has received, at least from a phenomenological perspective, some attention in the MS population too. A detailed, structured psychiatric interview was undertaken on 100 consecutive MS clinic attendees and revealed 17 people with major depression and almost three times as many with subsyndromal depression.[70] A comparison of these two groups showed comparable levels of overall psychological distress. Similar findings have emerged in the general psychiatry literature as well.[71,72] The following case history illustrates the challenges posed by such a situation and the benefits that come with treatment.

José is 45 years of age. He is married and has a 12-year-old daughter. He has an EDSS of 5.0 and can no longer work as a mechanic. He is a large man, with a fleshy, cherubic face. He is soft spoken and courteous. When we shake hands, my hand disappears into a giant mitt that still bears the telltale grease stains of his earlier work life. He is dressed neatly in jeans and a pressed T-shirt, which has the logo of his favorite football team, Real Madrid. He smiles easily and denies feeling depressed, notwithstanding the referral from his neurologist for a mood assessment. The most he admits to is a sense of heightened frustration at his failing physical health. Walking is now more difficult, fatigue is a bother, and eyesight is not so great. Sleep is impaired, appetite has increased, with some weight gain, but his enjoyment at watching football on TV, his main passion, is still intact. José does, however, shift a little uneasily when I bring the subject back to his mood, and it is clear to me he would rather talk about his beloved Real Madrid and the respective merits of Cristiano Ronaldo versus Lionel Messi. I ask how he might deal with his frustration. José shrugs his shoulders. "What is a man to do when he can no longer work?" he asks rhetorically. "Watch some more TV, go for a drive." He folds his arms defensively across a barrel chest and smiles benignly.

José gives me permission to speak with his wife. Maria is less than half her husband's size. She, too, is neatly groomed and soft spoken, but she looks troubled. To break the ice, I ask if she also likes Real Madrid. She smiles wanly and tells me there is no time for such things. A full-time job, a child on the cusp of becoming a teenager, a home to run, a disabled husband, the family budget under strain: who has time for sports? Clearly José does, and that is no doubt a source of some family tension, but rather than explore that dynamic for now, I ask her about her husband's mood. She hesitates before replying and reaches out for his arm. "I love my husband," she prefaces, before pausing. "I want him to be happy. We all want him to be happy. But now he is so angry we are scared of him." She falls silent and stares at the floor.

I have my opening and shift the question back to José. "Perhaps you would like to comment on what your wife has just said?" I inquire. He shrugs again, gives an awkward smile, and acknowledges that from time to time he feels upset. "And then what?" I ask. "How do you behave when you're upset?" "Sometimes I shout," admits José, looking sheepish. "Does it ever go beyond shouting?" I ask him. "Never," comes his instant response, and his wife nods in agreement.

The rest of the appointment is spent teasing out what makes José angry. Two conflicting accounts emerge: José playing down his temper and his wife repeating that she and their daughter are scared of his rages. "Has it always been this way?" I ask. Here, husband and wife are in agreement. Both believe that things changed about a year back when José had his most serious relapse, one that put an end to his work and left him unsteady on his feet. The session ends with Maria pushing for treatment and José brushing her off.

Two weeks later my secretary puts a call through to my office. It is from José's sister, and she sounds scared. She is calling from José's house, she informs me in a whisper, where she, Maria, and the couple's 12-year-old daughter have taken refuge in the bathroom. In the background, I hear José bellowing. The call is interrupted when the police arrive. A week later, José and Maria come to see me. Charges have not been laid, but it is clear that the arrival of two police officers has had a sobering effect on José's assessment of his home situation. Perhaps help is needed after all, he admits.

Two options are offered: medication or a referral to a men's anger-management group. José hurriedly chooses the first one. Talk therapy is not his strong point, he divulges. I hand out a prescription for an SSRI, after going through the benefits and potential side effects of treatment with him. Ten days later, Maria calls to thank me. She has her José back. Gone are the verbal explosions. No longer must she and her child walk on eggshells. Those paroxysms of rage that came out of nowhere, that were impossible to predict, that seemed so random and hurtful and out of keeping with her gentle giant's character are now gone. "Completely?" I ask. Maria hesitates. "Well almost completely," she divulges. "Except now it's different." There have been one or two times when she has seen the anger bubble, but then it just as quickly subsides. "Like a soufflé that goes poof!" is how she describes it to me. I am startled by her evocative metaphor for, try as I might, I cannot reconcile José's presence with a delicate soufflé. The more docile demeanor is certainly good news, however, and something that I can confirm in person at José's next appointment, when not only Maria accompanies him but his sister does too. The drug is a miracle, they chorus. Amidst profuse thanks, the two women hand over some pastries and a liter of homemade red wine. What José makes of proceedings is more difficult to discern. He sits there heavily, smiling benignly and every now and then shrugs his massive shoulders as if to infer, "Whatever!"

José's response to an SSRI was dramatic but not unusual. Antidepressant drugs are often effective when treating irritability, particularly if the behavioral change is linked to the neurological disorder. Far more intractable is the problem of irritability that long predates the MS diagnosis, with MS possibly exacerbating the problem. Here, the anger owes more to innate character, which brings to mind American football coach Doug Plank's witty observation that temperament in his players was 90% temper and 10% mental. When such a ratio is integral to a person's personality, a pill taken with breakfast is unlikely to give the desired therapeutic result.

Another interesting observation is that when irritability responds to an SSRI, an SNRI, or a tricyclic antidepressant, it can do so quickly. Improvement can be seen within 48–72 hours of starting treatment, significantly shorter than the lag time that comes with treating major depression using the same drugs. Supporting data for this observation comes from studies of irritability in people with traumatic brain injury,[73] premenstrual dysphoria,[74] and smoking cessation.[75] Reasons for this are unclear. The most parsimonious explanation may be that irritability is a single symptom, whereas major depression is a syndrome consisting of multiple symptoms, which collectively come with their own timeline for improvement.

[EIGHT]

More on Depression and the Causal Complexities of Enduring Sadness

THE PSYCHOSOCIAL LITERATURE exploring links with depression in people with multiple sclerosis is large and varied. We have already seen in Roza's case how a poor coping strategy like avoidance can fuel depression and leave a person mired in unhappiness. In addition, the coping literature tells us that aspects of emotion-based coping can prove problematic. Here, decisions are driven by heightened feelings of despair, frustration, irritability, and hopelessness. Emotion-driven decisions tend to be impulsive, sudden, poorly planned, and adopted in the mistaken belief that they will reduce the distress felt at the time. In the short term, these decisions may indeed have the desired effect, but benefits can prove transient and will be replaced by more enduring adverse consequences. An example of this maladaptive coping style is revealed in the following case history.

Jenna is 32 years of age and single. Ten years of multiple sclerosis have put an end to her international career as a model. Some work still comes her way, but through a different channel—a modeling agency for people with disabilities. "Not quite the same thing as before," she tearfully informs me. "Before my MS, I could hop on a plan and a few hours later begin a shoot in the Caribbean. And from there I could skip off to

Italy for another gig before jetting off to Hong Kong. That's how it was—a whirlwind of activity, cool places, good money, and my image in glossy, expensive magazines—a face that was known everywhere and, dare I say it, a body that turned heads. All gone now! Kaput!"

Her physical disability is profound. Cerebellar involvement has played havoc with her gait and coordination. Even a simple task like drinking coffee has become difficult. "Gone is my morning espresso," Jenna tells me. She cannot coordinate picking up such a tiny cup, and even should she eventually get her wayward hand to grasp it—forget about negotiating the handle—the path from saucer to lips is so jerky that the hot liquid flies everywhere, and with it comes the risk of scalding. "Imagine that, burning my face!" she exclaims. "The only part of my signature identity left untouched by my fucking disease!"

Jenna's low mood is inextricably linked to her physical disability. For much of her life her identity has been defined by her looks. Ever since adolescence, when it gradually dawned on her that people considered her beautiful, she traded on what she saw as her greatest asset to get what she wanted. She learned young that her appearance opened doors for her. She is frank in telling me how she manipulated her male teachers with a disarming smile, how she used a little seduction to gain access to a leading modeling agency, and how she had never been short of boyfriends and suitors. "You would not believe the gifts that came my way," she tells me. "Flowers, jewelry, business-class plane tickets, even a plasma TV . . . it was ridiculous. Often, I didn't even recognize the name on the card. Anyway, I always returned the gifts, except the flowers of course. I didn't want to be beholden."

Her modeling career took flight while she was still a student. She never completed high school. "Who needed a musty classroom when my workplaces were the beaches of Turks and Caicos or the French Riviera?" She was an only child. She had never been close to her distant parents. There was no pull of family. There was no best friend—no real friends at all. It had been easy to wave a premature goodbye to childhood and the few local connections made, walk out of home with all she ever needed in a Louis Vuitton suitcase, and assume a new identity elsewhere—live the cosmopolitan existence and pop back every now and then to a rented studio apartment in downtown Toronto to catch up on laundry and sleep before jetting off again. She recalls being so busy she never even had time to spend the good money that came her way.

When her MS first presented, she remembers thinking, amidst a flood of tears, that her time was limited now. As she saw it, a wheelchair beckoned and the clock was ticking. That meant cramming in even more work, never saying no to whatever new offer came her way, running as hard as she could to keep one step ahead of what she was convinced was a looming catastrophe. Every decision made was swayed by her sharpened emotions. She recalls her conviction that now was not the time to pause, reflect, plan, or heed what she saw was the unwanted fatherly advice of her neurologist. "What the hell do you know of life?" she recollects admonishing him. She was 22 years of age at the time.

To begin with, her plan seemed to work. Her initial symptoms faded, and she had no difficulty hitting her stride. She never divulged her diagnosis. "That would have been the kiss of death for my career," she informed me. "It's so damn competitive—one little chink in your armor and you're done for." She dealt with her first relapse by pleading exhaustion, certainly a plausible excuse given the pace of her career, and within two weeks she was back on the runway. But gradually, remorselessly, her cerebellar signs worsened. They could not always be hidden. "At first people thought I was drunk," she divulged. "You know, I would spill something, or stumble, or appear a little unsteady. And I would laugh along with all those little shits because it was much easier to pretend I was pissed or hungover than to divulge I had multiple sclerosis."

A worsening intention tremor, however, finally unmasked Jenna's secret. She recalled the moment with eidetic clarity. "There I was, in my agent's office, ready to sign the biggest contract of my career—a major solo shoot for Vogue. What a dream! The whole office so excited for me and for themselves, but when it came to sign, I couldn't hit the line. I just could not get the pen to come down on the dotted line. I fucked up my signature—it came out like spaghetti. I remember my agent saying, 'Easy Jen, no need to get so excited.' He was laughing, but nervously, and his secretary printed out another clean copy for me to sign, and the exact same thing happened again. Everyone was staring at me now, like horrified. It was 10 a.m. The sun was streaming in through the windows. The room was so damn hot, and I was sweating. I couldn't claim to be pissed. Not at 10 a.m."

A signature of sorts was obtained, but everything began unraveling quickly after that. The photo shoot had to be abandoned halfway through. "I couldn't keep my balance," Jenna recalled, "and the situation became dangerous because part of the shoot was on a yacht out at sea, and there was a real concern I would fall overboard. Abandoning the project was a nightmare. I could see everyone was furious at me, at the time lost, and at the money wasted, and there was nothing to show for it."

Keeping the diagnosis a secret was no longer an option. She broke the news tearfully to her agent. Her disclosure was greeted with shock but not surprise by those who knew her. "Everyone knew something had been wrong for some time," Jenna recollected, "and rumors spread quickly. But when the diagnosis was let out the bag, people in the industry understood the problem was bigger than they first thought." There was an outpouring of sympathy. Telephone calls, texts, cards, and flowers followed. Two weeks of good wishes, love, and support came her way. And then the world as she knew it moved on without her, hardly skipping a beat. Left alone in her sparsely furnished studio apartment with a waterfront view and the extravagant "get well" floral arrangements turning limp, she had ample time to take stock of a life that had come off the rails. Her neurologist was urging her to restart a disease-modifying drug, but Jenna remembered the side effects from her first trial: the skin at the injection site turning blue and darkening, with the swelling giving way to hard, painful lumps that looked unsightly. In a world in which appearance was everything, where the camera defined your reality, such disfigurement was potentially ruinous. Jenna shuddered as she recalled exposing her bruises to the gimlet eye of Erich, a legendary fashion photographer she had loved working with. He knew how to make her feel good, natural. He knew how to bring out the best in her with his smooth mix of friendly, funny banter, sexy talk, and cooing blandishments. They were in Dubrovnik, Croatia, an exquisite backdrop to a beautiful spring day, and as she stripped to her expensive lingerie (which she was being paid an embarrassing amount of money to show off), she saw his eyes widen in horror. "Holy shit, Jenna!" she remembers him exclaiming. "Were you hit by a bus?" She remembers Erich putting his camera aside and approaching her to take a closer look, and how she recoiled when he reached out his hand and gently ran it over one of those ugly, painful lumps, and how, sensing her pain, he had taken her head in his hands, looked her squarely in the eyes, and in that soothing voice of his reassured her that everything would be okay, 100% okay, because he was going to kill the son of a bitch who had done this to her.

Erich's threat had broken the tension and made her giggle. She recollects calling him a silly fool. Now it was his turn to appear hurt. The bruises, she informed him, were the unfortunate side effect of a medication. He looked skeptical. "Medication?" he queried. "What medication? You're as fit as a fiddle." "Allergy medication," she lied. Mollified, Erich picked up his camera. They worked well together over the next few days. Photoshop took care of the unsightly blemishes. On her last night in Dubrovnik, Jenna went for a midnight walk along the beach promenade and dumped her remaining medication, syringes, and needles in a garbage bin. Good riddance to a treatment that felt worse than the disease.

Two years later, alone in her apartment, her phone silent now, Jenna regretted her earlier impulsivity. There had been some work after Dubrovnik, but her modeling world had shrunk alarmingly since then. Catwalk work was out. She couldn't pull it off. "You know, the kind of fast-paced walk where you place one leg in front of the other, keeping a dead straight line," she explained, "so that your hips swing back and forth. When I tried that, I fell over. Definitely not a good advertisement for the couturier!" And then there was the challenge presented by high heels. "Stilettos had become my trapeze," she divulged, "and there was no safety net to catch me."

Jenna paused and looked wistfully out my ground-floor office window. For much of the year, it is not much of a view. A courtyard, open to one side, encloses some unruly grass, tenacious weeds, and a lone, untended sugar maple tree. But come the fall, the tree puts on a spectacular show, the foliage turning a vibrant reddish-orange that is offset to perfection by the surrounding dark brickwork. It was now late September, and on this cloudless, chilly day, the maple was in full fall foliage. "How lovely," she murmured to herself, her gaze arrested by the blaze of color. She fell silent, a shaft of late afternoon sunlight falling across her finely chiseled features, the subtle interplay of light and shadow accentuating her melancholy with Caravaggio-like effect.

When she spoke again, the spell of the moment was broken and replaced by bitter, hard words that cut to the very core of her despair. Stilettos now took center stage, the spiky, high heels a metaphor for what she had lost with this "damned" disease. "If you could give me one wish today, do you know what it would be?" she asked defiantly, no answer expected because in the very same breath she launched into a tearful tirade. "Well, let me tell you. One simple thing. One very, very simple thing. Let me get back into my stilettos without falling over. Let me walk in my stilettos the way I once could. To feel that walk again, to experience what it means to me, how good it makes me feel, the confidence I have with that walk, knowing the looks I get, the admiration—I feel like a queen on high. You have no idea how good that makes me feel. Silly, isn't it? Just a pair of shoes, really, but it comes with so much more. With that walk, in those shoes, it doesn't matter that I dropped out of school. That walk gives me far more that math, civics, and English ever can. Those shoes open career doors, fill my bank account, and send men scurrying after me, tripping over their gifts. When I put on my favorite pair, I am in charge of my life. They are my passport. Oh, yes, they are! Something special."

In the months ahead, with her career on the skids, Jenna would return to her stiletto talk repeatedly. It was as though she was trying to bargain with fate, reach some agreement with the mysterious, unknown forces that controlled her illness. "Just grant me one thing," she would beseech. "Just one request. Not much to ask, is it? To walk in my stilettos again!" Her pleas were accompanied by tears and racking sobs. She angrily refused all medication. Antidepressants would make her fat and hypnotics would make her an addict, she complained. Her window for obtaining benefits from a disease-modifying drug had passed because she had entered a secondary progressive disease course a decade before ocrelizumab, siponimod, and rituximab would emerge as treatments for people with progressive forms of MS.[1-3]

Talk therapy centered on trying to manage Jenna's unrealistic expectations and curtail her emotional venting. Asking heatedly and repeatedly for something that was unattainable meant constant disappointment and, with it, despondency and despair. It was also so much easier now to live in the past, clinging to memories of her face and body filling the pages of heavy, glossy magazines, the comfort of business-class travel, the allure of beautiful beaches and glitzy hotels, and the admiration and respect and love that flowed her way from agents, photographers, colleagues, and yes, even strangers. How wonderful it had all been. The comforting glow of nostalgia skipped over the exhaustion of constant travel, the vicious backstabbing jealousy, the hassle of having to constantly watch your weight, the anxiety of knowing that careers were often short because age could not be held indefinitely at bay. Living in the past offered far more than rose-tinted memories. Avoidance coupled with warm emotion-laden memories from her glamorous past now dulled the pain of the present. It also hindered coming to terms with illness and disability and planning for the future.

A new difficulty surfaced in therapy, one that was also emotion-driven. Jenna's complicated love life. MS had deprived her of much, but it had not taken away her looks. A damaged cerebellum had destroyed her coordination, but like Roza, whose dysfunctional pyramidal tracts made walking so labored, when Jenna remained still there were no outward signs of the disease. Sitting quietly at a table in a café kept a connection of sorts to the world around her. Heads still turned to look at her. She knew it and exulted in it, just as she knew it would be devastating to try and lift the cup to her lips because how many times had she seen a look of admiration or flirtation turn to stunned surprise and then pity as her wayward hand flapped uncontrollably. So there she sat, unmoving, sphinx-like, every now and then her helper leaning over discretely with a bottle of mineral water for Jenna to drink with a straw.

The siren song of her looks still pulled in would-be suitors, but most fled when confronted by her disability. Those who stayed differed from the men who had beaten a path to her door during happier days. The fast men with money and expensive designer shades gave way to the guy who delivered her groceries, the driver who ferried her to medical appointments, and the handyman who replaced the light bulbs. Extravagant floral arrangements were supplanted by modest posies as a marker of courtship. Jenna, for all her emotional pain, enjoyed these dalliances and was skillful in ensuring that none of her would-be suitors bumped into one another unexpectedly. But her happiness here was fleeting, the rendezvous organized as a brief pick-me-up. All her decisions and plans were driven by her emotions in the moment. There were no well-thought-out strategies to offset her disability, no calm reflection on what was needed for her future. Instead, impulsivity allied to an emotional lability dictated her path through a rapidly shrinking lifestyle. She was profligate with money, buying some luxury item hardly needed for the feel-good effect that was quickly lost as counterweight to her physical disability. She appeared incapable of letting go of the past, against which every present thought, feeling, and action was measured. Her wheelchair tormented her, viewed with shame and loathing, the antithesis of her stilettos. As to the stilettos, she refused to sell them or give them away. Instead, they occupied pride of place in her walk-in closet, trophies of past success, and a constant reminder of what was no longer attainable.

As I got to know Jenna better during her weekly therapy sessions, it became clear that even before the onset of her MS she had been an emotional person. Decisions had been made quickly, albeit shrewdly when it came to her professional life. She had thrived on the excitement of a jet-setting lifestyle and a tempestuous bohemian life. Relationships had been fraught, explosive at times. There were few shades of gray in how she saw people. Those she met were quickly classified as either wonderful or terrible, geniuses or idiots, gorgeous or ugly, generous or miserly, and so on. When she could see that her initial assessment had been incorrect, she self-corrected by quickly shifting to the opposite extreme. These wild swings in judgment had not been conducive to building good, lasting friendships. Indeed, there had been little time for friendships in general given her pace of life. "Who needed them?" she dismissively asked. "Work and travel filled my days. There was no time for any-thing else. Oh yes, a quick fling here or there, and then I was off to the next destination."

Now, 10 years of multiple sclerosis had brought Jenna's life to a very different place. What had not changed, however, was an approach to life and relationships driven by her emotions. If anything, the MS had intensified this trait. Change would entail a lot of therapy, hard intro-spective work, and the capacity for delayed gratification. None of this came easy to her. Her waning reserves of energy were spent trying to make the moment more emotionally comfortable. These short-term fixes entailed living in the past, recalling happy memories as a substitute for present despair, impulse shopping, and seducing the delivery men who entered her shrinking world. Advice, medical or otherwise, that did not immediately take the sting out of her current distress was angrily and tearfully dismissed.

When Jenna was riding high in her career, she could get by with her emotion-driven coping style. Those around her cut her a lot of slack. Success can do this, establishing a different set of ground rules by which behavior is judged. Now that she was using a wheelchair and was de-pendent on caregivers to bathe, dress, and feed her, the power differen-tial had shifted in her relationships. For the first time in her adult life, Jenna needed people. This need was so desperate at times that it scared her. The challenge here was magnified by her loneliness. Time, that elu-sive commodity during the helter-skelter professional years, slowed to a crawl. As a model, she had lived 25-hour days. There had never been enough time. Now, courtesy of her MS, there was too much of it. Alone in her apartment, marooned by her illness, Jenna had a sense of time slowing. Her caregivers came early to get her out of bed and set her up for the day. By 9 a.m. they were gone, and the day stretched out end-lessly in front of her. Someone would pop in around midday to help with lunch, which she never ate anyway, her bird-like appetite a throw-back to her modeling days. Then the morning ritual would be repeated in the evening, but in reverse order this time, when the team returned to prepare her for the night. By nine in the evening, she had been fed, washed, and tucked into bed with nothing but insomnia to look forward to. From time to time, one of her boyfriends would spend an evening with her or a caregiver would take her out to a café, breaking the monotony of an existence in which the days blurred into one another, weekends lost their meaning, and only the passing of the seasons marked her calendar.

So much time now! Sitting alone in her still, quiet apartment waiting for time to pass. "To what end?" she asked herself. The answer was too painful to contemplate. The phone seldom rang. The speed with which she had lost contact with her former life painfully unmasked a truth that she had been unaware of. She had no friends. Agents, fellow models, photographers, favorite maître d's, travel agents, and that whole coterie of hangers-on who had always greeted her so effusively with extravagant compliments were revealed for who they had always been. Illness ruthlessly striped away any illusions. As for her parents, well they were old now and seemed just as overwhelmed by their daughter's disability as she was. Their uncertainty offered no comfort, just more irritation. With so much time to mull things over, Jenna could see all too clearly that she was quite alone now. She had never been someone comfortable only in her company. She had always avoided being alone. Which made it all the harder now to sit day after day in a wheelchair looking out a window at the placid lake in an apartment so still you could hear the faint, relentless ticking of the kitchen clock.

Emotions still ruled her decisions. Her treating team had a number of suggestions to lessen her isolation. Jenna rejected them all. Swimming entailed being undressed in a public changing room, humiliating in itself, and then essentially being carried into the shallow end of a highly chlorinated, uncomfortably warm indoor pool, where she would be deposited under the watchful eye of a rehabilitation support worker, just like a baby, and allowed to stand unassisted until the whistle was blown and it was time to go home. How could that compare to sunning herself on white sands and plunging into the azure waters of the Caribbean to cool off? The same cutting view was taken of the weekly support groups offered. How could sitting in a circle with eight people in wheelchairs, all old enough to be her parents—in some case grandparents—and talking about how life had dealt them all a bad hand compare with those delicious moments around some far-off bar, rubbing shoulders with young, beautifully honed bodies in the full bloom of youth? And then there were those dreadful bingo evenings, bused off to some tired community center for an evening of what she saw as enforced jollity. Her helper would sit alongside her marking the card, and she recalls with mortification the one evening when she won: the excited hollering of "BINGO!" by her helper, all the wheelchairs in the hall swiveling so that their occupants could see who had won, and her discomfort at the congratulations that came her way. Rather than soak up the moment of good cheer, of solidarity genuinely expressed, all she could think of was a warm summer's night in Deauville, France, a couple of years back when she had placed all her chips on number 1 and the roulette ball had run in her favor, and as a "shit pile" of chips was shoveled in her direction, she had overheard someone say "to beauty goes the spoils."

There you have it, the nub of Jenna's problem. Every aspect of her life now was compared to life before the onset of illness—the differences viewed in extremes. In reality, the contrast was marked, for her disability by now was severe, and yet it was just as evident that her tendency to denigrate what was now on offer to her was self-defeating. Unable to reign in her emotions, she preferred reliving past triumphs, cocooned in memories that temporarily assuaged the pain of loss even as they hindered future planning and paradoxically left her more vulnerable to the debilitating effects of her depression. I wish I could report a happier outcome here. Therapy at best proved marginally palliative.

The maladaptive coping strategies described thus far, predominantly avoidant in Roza's case and emotion focused but also encompassing avoidance with Jenna, are not all-or-none phenomena. Not every aspect of their responses to the challenges presented by their MS betrayed poor decision making. Similarly, the reader will recognize at times the overlap between avoidance and emotion-driven responses. Clean-cut divisions are typically more the preserve of case histories written to illustrate a particular point than a reflection of the complexities of clinical practice. Individuals most often display an array of responses that, in some cases, might tilt toward avoidance and in others be more emotion based. And interspersed among these are to be found healthier, more adaptive strategies as well. This mix will vary from person to person and, like every other behavioral attribute described in this book, will fall along a continuum.

In addition, while the emphasis in this chapter is on depression and the factors that leave an individual more vulnerable to it, there are other comorbid difficulties that cannot be overlooked in assessing the individual and planning the appropriate interventions. Both Roza and Jenna had entered a secondary progressive disease phase where the likelihood of cognitive dysfunction increases. Both women did indeed have problems with processing speed and memory, and in Roza's case, executive challenges too. While it is important to emphasize that avoidance and emotion-based coping strategies are not inextricably bound up with faulty cognition, these intellectual stumbling blocks can exert a negative effect on coping strategies, as mentioned earlier.[4] Furthermore, there are data showing that impaired cognition more than total brain lesion volume can influence the effectiveness of therapy for depression in people with MS.[5] Recall the study in which cognitive behavior therapy (CBT), supportive-expressive group therapy, and sertraline were compared as treatments for depression.[6] MRI and neuropsychological testing were given to a subset of participants. Six months following completion of treatment, scores on the Beck Depression Inventory for the entire sample were predicted by neuropsychological performance only. While total lesion volume predicted cognitive performance, it did not do the same for depression. Cognition therefore appeared to mediate the effects of therapy for depression, an intriguing finding that awaits replication.

Now that we've seen the degree to which mood suffers when individuals respond to their MS-related disability in dysfunctional ways, let us change gears and explore the upside of a different response to the disease. The positive effects of problem-focused coping are highlighted in the following case report. Meera is 42 years of age, single, and lives alone. She formerly worked as an insurance adjuster, but impaired mobility and fatigue put an end to her career. Eighteen years of MS have left her using a wheelchair. Like Roza and Jenna, Meera has entered a secondary progressive disease phase. But this is where the similarities end.

Meera finds structure helpful to her emotional well-being. She plans her days in advance, conscious of the need to balance her activities with the periods of rest her fatigue demands. She has accepted that many of the activities she formerly enjoyed are now beyond her: working in a fast-paced office, going for a jog, putting on gourmet dinner parties for friends, hiking the mountain trails of Alberta and British Columbia. However, she has compensated for these losses in a number of ways. To begin with, she replaced her car with a van that was capable of comfortably accommodating a wheelchair. She can self-load the wheelchair into the van, where it locks in place, and from there she transfers to the driver's seat. Hand controls have been installed for the gas and brakes. She has retaken her driver's test in the modified van and is now licensed to drive. Guaranteeing her own mobility in this way was a big boost to her self-confidence and self-esteem. She described her first drive in her newly equipped van as "completely liberating, a game changer."

When it came to entertaining, Meera hit on an original idea. She would keep the dinner parties going. She loved them and so did her friends, but recognizing her limitations, she could no longer spend the day preparing three courses for her guests. Her solution was to shift some of the preparation onto those attending. She would buy all the ingredients, but one couple would be set the task of organizing the starter while another couple would oversee the entrée. Nothing too complicated here—gone were the days of her signature bouillabaisse, and desserts were now bought rather than concocted from elaborate recipes. She supplied the wine and liqueurs, generous quantities of which lubricated the evenings nicely, she confided.

As for her love of travel, that too was satisfied, albeit within the limitations of her disease. She traveled to Los Angeles often to keep alive a long-distance relationship. She made sure the airline company knew of her disability well in advance of her departure date and was delighted to find how accommodating they were, assisting her in navigating the complexities of the airport with minimal fuss.

Exercise was also part of her daily routine. A physiotherapist would come to her home weekly and set a program for her, much of it based on her intact upper limb abilities. Exercise and a little massage did wonders for how she was feeling, both physically and emotionally, she reported. But the cherry on the cake of all her activities, the one that confirmed—if confirmation was ever needed—that she retained her "mojo" were her biannual half-marathons in which she propelled herself through the streets of Toronto and Boston in her manual streamlined wheelchair. She kept a photo album of her multiple marathons—a visual record of exhaustion and exhilaration.

Meera's mental state was interesting. While her mood was generally good, she was not consistently chipper and upbeat. Her resolve and careful planning did not negate the distress that came from an unyielding, debilitating disease that intruded into every aspect of her daily life. She would never leave her wheelchair. Pain was tenaciously persistent. Fatigue set a daily ambush. Memory would embarrass her from time to time. All around her, life hurried on while she struggled to keep up. She saw how easily her friends walked, ran, bent over, straightened up, squatted, twisted, turned, pivoted, arose effortlessly from a chair and settled gently into one, and danced, jumped, and pirouetted on the dance floor, all without second thought—movements she would never again be able to perform. She never resented this, never begrudged her friends their robust health, even if they took if for granted. Instead, she quietly, privately mourned what she had lost while keeping her focus on what needed to be done to offset her limitations.

Meera's life is an affirmation of what can be achieved by someone with a significant disability. She did not live in the past. She did not bemoan her fate. She was an effective planner and spent much of her time, energy, and financial resources realizing her plans. Her sadness was invariably transient. She had never needed antidepressant medication or CBT. She had learned how to cope with her illness, how to adapt her life's circumstances to her disability. She did not avoid the challenges that could so easily clog the way forward. Decisions were not driven by the emotions of the moment but instead carefully thought through and, where possible, executed. Such an approach was not just dependent on innate temperament. It also required intact cognition. Apart from some mild deficits in learning and memory, her intellectual abilities had fortunately been spared. What was notable about her approach was that it came from within her. Psychotherapy may have helped fine-tune some of the strategies, but that was all it had to offer. She had essentially found the solution to living well with MS herself. In this regard Meera became a role model for others. This does not imply that everything she did was suitable for everyone. Half-marathons twice a year were a personal challenge, an affirmation of fortitude, endurance and will power that worked for her. For others, the mere thought of such exertions would be overwhelming. It was Meera's mental approach to her disease rather than the specific nature of her actions that offered the template to follow.

In the case histories of Roza, Jenna, and Meera, the focus has been on the coping mechanisms that either protect against depression or leave people vulnerable to it. All three women were significantly disabled but only Meera was able to look past her physical limitations and embrace a way of life that remained rich and varied. Here she was aided by her minimal cognitive compromise. Not surprisingly, she was the one who never developed depression. The triad of physical disability, coping style, and depression therefore offers a plausible explanation for why depression may arise in some people, and it also offers a useful starting point for therapy. Helpful as this is, however, it is only part of the etiological conundrum of depression in people with MS. This point is underscored by some studies,[7,8] but not others,[9,10] reporting an association between depression and physical disability. This too should not come as a surprise. The complexities of depression currently defy a single etiological explanation. Important as coping strategies are, we need to broaden our field of inquiry if we are to understand these complexities more fully.

Let me start by briefly refuting two potential causes of depression and promoting a third. There are no compelling findings that point to a shared genetic predisposition to MS and depression,[9,11,12] despite the occasional dissenting voice.[13] There is also no consistent data attributing depression to disease-modifying therapy. An early scare arose with publication of the first disease-modifying-therapy trial, which revealed that four people receiving interferon beta-1β attempted suicide and one died by suicide, in comparison with no such outcomes in the placebo group.[14,15] Subsequent reports seemed to confirm that depression could arise with treatment.[16,17] However, as data accumulated over time, it became clearer that depression following treatment with one of the interferon drugs was not a specific drug-related side effect[18,19] but rather was associated with depression pretreatment and unrealistic expectations of treatment.[20,21] Furthermore, a recent systemic review, while failing to find compelling evidence of depression as a side effect of treatment, actually concluded that one of the disease-modifying therapies—namely, fingolimod—improved depression.[22] This consensus has been challenged recently by the findings from a German cohort study of over 15,000 people treated with a disease-modifying drug between 2006 and 2013.[23] The most frequent serious adverse side effect of treatment documented was admission to hospital with depression. There were no differences in rates of depression across different disease-modifying therapies. This finding, however, should be seen within the context of depression being common in people with MS to begin with. As noted earlier, findings from a large community study revealed that one in four people with MS is likely to develop depression over the course of a year.[24] Furthermore, some of the studies reporting a high prevalence of depression long predate the arrival of disease-modifying treatments.[11,25] Nevertheless, given that group data can obscure individual susceptibilities, a cautious view holds that every person with MS who begins disease-modifying treatment should be monitored for changes in mood. Then again, this recommendation holds true for everyone with MS.

Now that we have largely ruled out genetic factors and disease-modifying therapy in our quest to understand the origins of MS-related depression, let us shift our focus to neuroinflammation. We know that MS is an inflammatory disease. There is also evidence, unrelated to MS, suggesting that symptoms of mental illness, such as depression, anxiety, mania, and psychosis, are mediated by inflammatory processes.[26,27] It is therefore reasonable to assume the same for people with MS who become depressed and anxious. Surprisingly, the literature exploring this fertile topic in MS is very small. However, a recent study of 405 people with relapsing-remitting MS has given the inflammatory theory a much needed boost.[28] Brain MRIs with contrast enhancement were obtained at baseline and at six months thereafter. Active disease was defined by clinical relapse or signs of disease activity on contrast enhanced MRI. In addition, cerebrospinal fluid was available from a subset of 111 treatment-naïve participants, from which concentrations of a number of pro-inflammatory cytokines were obtained. These included inter-leukin (IL) -1β, IL-2, IL-8, tumor necrosis factor–α (TNF-α), and interferon-Υ. Higher levels of depression and state, not trait, anxiety were found in radiologically active individuals, with symptoms decreasing as brain inflammation resolved. Of note is that steroids, a potent anti-inflammatory agent given during relapses, reduced mood disturbances. Rounding out the inflammatory picture, associations were found between IL-2 and anxiety, and between IL-1β/TNF-α and depression. Significantly, anxiety was found to predict disease reactivation, an association explained on the basis of IL-2 being produced by T-cell activation. The study, apart from drawing attention to a neglected field of behavioral inquiry in people with MS, also raised some interesting clinical questions, such as the potential effectiveness of anti-inflammatory agents as a treatment for mood disorders in this group (the positive response to steroids leading the way) and, conversely, the potential benefits from psychotropic agents (such as antidepressant and antipsychotic medications) as disease-modifying therapies.

An interesting corollary to these findings are data showing a rising incidence in psychiatric disorders up to five years before the diagnosis of inflammatory diseases such as MS, inflammatory bowel disease, and rheumatoid arthritis.[29] Reasons for this remain unclear, perhaps reflecting shared risk factors for psychiatric illness and immune-mediated illness, a shared final, common inflammatory pathway, or another cause yet to be elucidated.

Intriguing as the inflammatory hypothesis is, the most compelling etiological clues to MS-related depression are to be found in neuroimaging. In the late 1980s and early 1990s, when neuropsychiatric research related to people with MS was energized by the advent of MRI, the search for brain-behavior associations began in earnest. The studies that focused on cognition were soon reporting correlations that linked impairment to total and regional lesion area. As the imaging analyses became more sophisticated, lesion area, a two-dimensional measurement, was replaced by three-dimensional volume estimations, and the strength of the correlations increased. Atrophy also emerged as an even more significant marker of cognitive dysfunction. No such consistent findings, however, were forthcoming from the early imaging studies of depression, where negative findings predominated. There were many reasons for this. Depression has a more complex etiology than cognitive decline that includes a host of potential psychosocial factors, as we have seen. Cognition, on the other hand, is firmly rooted in brain function and structure, and while there are recognized confounders of cognitive performance, such as pain, fatigue, and emotional distress,[30] a more reductionist approach to understanding causation is supported by the data.

A second reason for the absence of brain-behavior correlates in the early depression imaging studies pertained to the limitations of MRI at the time. A weak field strength and thick slice sequence meant that subtler brain abnormalities were missed. In the late 1980s, the standard MRI machine had a field strength of 0.15 tesla, and brain slices were typically 10 mm or more apart. Today, the standard MRI machine is 3.0 tesla, 20 times more powerful, and slice thickness has come down to 3 mm for clinical use and 1 mm for many research protocols. The first MRI machines may have been a quantum leap forward in visualizing the brain in vivo, but clues as to the cerebral origins of depression would have to wait for the technology to improve.

The breakthrough came in 1997. A Spanish group undertook an MRI study of 45 people with MS who were all asked to complete the Beck Depression Inventory.[31] The imaging analysis was still relatively unsophisticated given that lesion area not volume was quantified, but the result was nevertheless a revelation. The data showed that depression was associated with lesions in the left suprainsular white matter, a region that comprises the arcuate fasciculus. Significantly, this could account for 17% of the depression variance. Put another way, the regional brain pathology could explain, in part—a small part to be sure—why certain people with MS became depressed. Not every depressed person had lesions in the arcuate fasciculus, hence the modest variance. However, in general, as scores on the Beck Depression Inventory increased, so the lesion area in the arcuate fasciculus increased as well. What was less clear was why this region in particular should be considered important with respect to mood. After all, the arcuate fasciculus is not part of the limbic brain, those regions that are known to be implicated in depression. Rather, its function in the left hemisphere is linked to language processing. One possible explanation therefore is to look at connections, as the arcuate fasciculus is a broad band of white matter fibers that extends from the ventrolateral frontal cortex, via the parietal cortex, all the way into the middle and inferior temporal lobes.[32] It is here in these frontotemporal regions that connections with limbic structures occur.

In a subsequent report, Pujol et al.[33] undertook a factor analysis of their Beck data and broke it down into four groups: affective (mood) symptoms, somatic (bodily) complaints, performance difficulties, and cognitive distortions. They found that lesion area in the arcuate fasciculus could now account for 26% of the depression variance in the first two categories.

The first study that signaled the importance of cerebral atrophy as a potential marker of depression appeared three years after the lesion data.[34] The intensity of depression was now linked to focal atrophy in frontal regions and those surrounding the third and lateral ventricles. An association with lesion volume was also reported, but for hypointense lesions only, the "black holes" that reflect more destructive, degenerative, and irreversible brain changes. This coupled with the atrophy findings suggested that depression was related to more ominous evidence of brain pathology.

Four years later, my lab also published a paper showing that multiple MRI indices could shed light on the brain changes that accompany depression.[35] Unlike earlier studies, we did not rely on patients' self-report symptoms to assess mood, but instead we undertook a structured interview used to diagnose major depression. Furthermore, conscious of multiple psychosocial influences on mood, we adopted a case-control design in which we matched people with and without major depression not only demographically and cognitively but also on their degree of social support and stress. We thus had two MS groups, similar in every way but one—the presence or absence of a major depression. With such a design, we had confidence that any MRI differences between the groups could be explained by depression alone. Our results showed that the depressed group had significantly more limbic involvement—namely, higher hyperintense and hypointense lesion volumes in the medial inferior prefrontal cortex and more extensive atrophy in anterior temporal regions. Taken collectively, these imaging changes more than doubled the depression variance reported earlier by Pujol et al.[31]

Further evidence that brain pathology was implicated in depression came from a German study of 29 people with relapsing-remitting MS and 20 healthy participants.[36] The focus was on the hippocampus, which was finely imaged to reveal some of its components. Symptoms of depression were recorded with the Beck Depression Inventory–revised. The MRI data revealed the people with MS who were depressed had more atrophy of the dentate gyrus and hippocampal regions CA2 and CA3. But the authors did not stop there. Participants had their serum cortisol levels checked three times a day (8:00 a.m., 4:00 p.m., 9:00 p.m.) over two consecutive days. A long-standing biological theory holds that depression is associated with abnormal functioning of the hypothalamic-pituitary-adrenal axis. One manifestation of this is an elevated serum cortisol level that does not follow the normal circadian rhythm of high in the mornings and low at night. To a degree, this was found in the present study too. Cortisol, which is a stress hormone, can cause brain atrophy if concentrations are elevated, as they were here, but only in the depressed MS group. What the researchers also found was that the atrophy was selective, confined to specific areas of the hippocampus.

Lesions and atrophy are only part of the story, however. There are other MRI indices that give us information on the structural integrity of *normal-appearing* brain tissue. One such technique is diffusion tensor imaging (DTI) that measures water diffusion in at least six different directions within the brain, thereby detecting microstructural changes invisible to the naked eye. DTI metrics, such as mean diffusivity (MD), measure the overall diffusivity of the brain, while fractional anisotropy (FA) provides information on the degree of directional restriction of the diffusion of water. ("A Hitchhiker's Guide to Diffusion Tensor Imaging" by Soares et al. offers a detailed account of this imaging modality.)[37]

My lab undertook a DTI study of 62 people with MS, 30 of whom were depressed.[38] For our imaging analyses, we began by segmenting hyperintense and hypointense lesions and cerebral gray and white matter. Removing the lesions left normal-appearing brain tissue. The next step entailed obtaining FA and MD images of normal-appearing brain tissue, which were then parcellated into anatomical subdivision. The end result left us with FA and MD imaging maps of normal-appearing brain tissue divided into specific anatomical loci. Comparisons were then undertaken between depressed and nondepressed individuals. Once more, the depressed group was found to have more pathological changes—namely, reduced FA and elevated MD in anterior temporal and inferior frontal regions. When these changes from normal-appearing brain tissue were added to the greater lesion burden and more extensive atrophy seen in the depressed group, these cumulative pathological brain changes pushed the variance in accounting for depression close to 50%.

The imaging findings in depressed people with MS described so far have all been structural. These are complemented by functional MRI changes that reveal the networks that have become dysfunctional too. In an elegant study, Italian researchers selected a group of 12 people with MS without a history of depression or anxiety and a group of 12 healthy individuals matched for age and education.[39] While undergoing an MRI, participants were tasked with matching a series of images of unfamiliar faces according to their negative expressions of sadness, fear, or anger. In keeping with expectations, both groups activated their amygdala, ventrolateral prefrontal cortex (vlPFC), thalamus, and visual cortex—areas that are known to process sensory and emotionally salient stimuli. However, while the healthy control group showed *changes* in connectivity between the amygdala and the vlPFC and medial prefrontal cortex (mPFC) during the task, no such changes were seen the MS group.

This lack of connectivity was thought to underlie the enhanced activation seen in the vlPFC in the MS group and was interpreted as a compensatory mechanism geared toward limiting the clinical expression of emotional symptoms. What it also reveals is the "inefficiency" of the MS brain when processing emotional stimuli, an adaptive response that nevertheless may leave the individual at heightened risk for developing a depressive disorder.

Dysfunctional connectivity between the amygdala and the prefrontal cortex was also reported by Riccelli et al.,[40] who likewise used facial imagery of sadness and anger in a functional MRI study of 77 people with MS. Increasing levels of depressive symptoms were again associated with reduced connectivity between the amygdala and dorsolateral prefrontal cortex (dlPFC) and vlPFC and increased activation in the prefrontal areas. A similar pattern of reduced connectivity was also found between the hippocampus and orbitofrontal cortex (OFC) with concomitant increased activation in the latter. Of note is that these dysfunctional connections between the amygdala and hippocampus, on the one hand, and prefrontal areas such as the dlPFC, vlPFC, and OFC, on the other, are supported structurally by the results of a DTI study showing an increase in path length between these very same regions.[41] Intriguingly, increased path lengths were also present with respect to connections to the motor-sensory cortex and supplementary motor regions, with the authors suggesting that these limbic-motor disturbances could have implications for the emotions that drive survival-oriented behaviors.

The neuroimaging findings in the MS depression literature confirm the importance of limbic pathology. But marrying the clinical, imaging, and therapeutic data can prove challenging. For example, the theoretical benefits of stress management were graphically illustrated in a 48-week neuroimaging study of 121 people with MS randomized to either a cognitive behavioral stress management group or a wait-list control group.[42] Treatment was provided for 16 sessions over 20–24 weeks, with all participants followed for another 24 weeks. MRI with contrast enhancement was undertaken at baseline and thereafter every eight

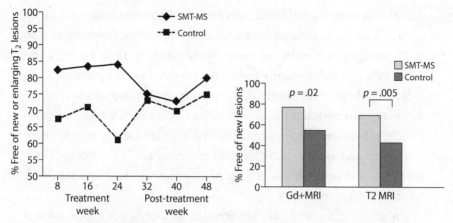

Figure 8.1. The time-limited effects of stress management therapy (SMT) on MRI metrics of disease activity in people with MS. Gd = Gadolinium (contrast enhanced). See ref. 42 in chap. 8.

weeks for the duration of the trial. The results showed that those individuals who received stress management acquired fewer contrast enhancing lesions, indicative of active disease, and fewer new lesions in general, but only during the period of receiving the intervention. No sooner had the intervention stopped than the MRI benefits were lost (figure 8.1). No clinical benefits accrued from the stress intervention in terms of fewer disease exacerbations or improved neurological function. Unfortunately, and surprisingly, the authors did not include a measure of mental well-being in their clinical analysis.

The stress reduction-imaging data mesh with the results of a systematic review and meta-analysis of psychosocial interventions on immune system function, which confirmed the power of psychotherapy to influence biological markers of inflammation.[43] While only two of the 56 randomized controlled studies that met inclusion criteria were MS related, the overall implications for people with MS are equally applicable. Eight psychosocial interventions, weighted toward CBT but also including psychoeducation, bereavement, and supportive therapy, improved immune system function measured a number of different ways (e.g., proinflammatory cytokines, anti-inflammatory cytokines, antibody levels, immune cell counts, and natural killer cell activity, among others).

Relative to control conditions, active interventions were associated with a 14.7% improvement in beneficial immune system function and an 18% decrease in harmful immune system function. Benefits to the immune system, predominantly from CBT, persisted for at least six months following therapy cessation. This is an important observation from an MS perspective given the proven benefits of CBT in MS-related depression.[6,44] This therefore suggests that CBT-type treatments may be more advantageous than a stress reduction intervention in MS where improvements in disease activity noted on MRI (see figure 8.1) dissipate with treatment cessation.[42]

Enlightening as the MRI data are, they cannot as yet inform clinical practice. Here psychiatry lags behind neurology, where MRI now plays a central role in clinical decision making. The diagnosis of major depression remains a clinical one. The imaging data that differentiate depressed from nondepressed individuals are group data. Currently, MRI lacks the sensitivity to make this distinction at the individual level. Nevertheless, there is still a clinical utility to MRI in that the literature reinforces the relatively new construct of depression as a brain disease. In 1994, the old organic-functional divide was removed from the American Psychiatric Association's classification of mental illness with publication of the fourth edition of the *Diagnostic and Statistical Manual of Mental Disorders*.[45] Overnight the word "organic" was gone, for it was seen as harkening back to bygone eras that had entrenched a false dichotomy—namely, that some mental illnesses, such as dementia, but not others, such as depression, were associated with a perturbation in brain function. As psychiatry approached the millennium, the discipline at last felt confident in asserting that *all* mental illnesses were brain illnesses.

The same conclusions apply to understanding the origins of MS-related depression. Thinking of depression as a brain disorder does not negate the importance of coping strategies, resilience, or self-efficacy as factors that can contribute to depression and recovery from it. On the contrary, in my clinical experience, the MS imaging findings can prove useful in treating a depressed person. Here is one example: a 46-year-old woman with MS and no family history of depression now presents for the first time with six of the nine symptoms used to diagnose a major depression. Her Expanded Disability Status Scale (EDSS) score is 1.5, indicative of mild physical disability. She has a good job, a happy marriage, two healthy and smart children, and enough money in the bank to live well. She eschews avoidant and emotion-based coping. Her life, judged by all these external markers of success and well-being, is good. And yet she is depressed, and she would like to know why. It's a good question, and one that I am often called on to answer.

The first possibility is that she has two independent diseases: MS and depression. After all, both are common, and so their co-occurrence in her could be by chance. But we also know that major depression is much more common in people with MS than the general population, and so the likelihood of a causal association is high. In the absence of psychosocial stressors and a dysfunctional coping style, it is reasonable to reference the neuroimaging data and suggest that her depression is a direct consequence of her MS, a brain disease. Her MRI is abnormal, and even though there are no contrast enhancing lesions, a marker of active disease, it is plausible the widespread lesions observed have disrupted neural circuits transporting biogenic amines, such as serotonin and noradrenaline, that control mood.

An explanation like this, which can never be sold as an absolute to someone with MS given the limits to current knowledge, can nevertheless be reassuring to those with depression. Many people with MS want to know about their disease; they follow advances in neuroscience with a keen interest and, like clinicians and researchers in the field, are fascinated by new discoveries, fresh insights, and novel concepts. Taking the time to explain to people with MS where their depression may be coming from, an explanation that goes beyond abstractions by bringing in something concrete that can be visualized, like MR images, can be rewarding to the person and doctor alike. And for a depressed person with MS, it may help assuage guilt and self-blame, for individuals frequently view their depression as the consequence of something they have done wrong, a personal failing.

Before concluding the chapters on depression, I return to a point made earlier in this book. In a disease without cure, good symptom management is often the buffer to despair and hope abandoned. Nowhere is this more true than for depression. The illness by its very nature can entail despondency and a feeling that life has lost all meaning and enjoyment. Numerous studies have shown how depression is a major determinant of quality of life for a person with MS.[46,47] It may further compromise cognitive function, as we have seen. And now there is evidence it can increase neurological disability as well. A Swedish cohort study revealed that people with depression were at significantly higher risk of worsening EDSS scores, and the same was true for those individuals prescribed antidepressant medications.[48] The result was replicated in a retrospective Canadian cohort study of 2,312 people newly diagnosed with MS who had been followed for 10.5 years.[49] Approximately one-third of the cohort developed a depressive or anxiety disorder in this period and were found to have a higher EDSS once data were adjusted for age, sex, socioeconomic status, disease course and duration, physical comorbidity, and treatment with a disease-modifying therapy. This finding reached statistical significance for women only.

As noted above, three compelling factors underline the importance of depression in the lives of people with MS: a reduced quality of life and deteriorating neurological and cognitive functions. To these must be added a fourth, one linked directly to mortality. Compared to age- and sex-matched people in the general population, people with MS are twice as likely to die by suicide, and while not every suicide is driven by depression, many are.[50] As I have written previously, "There is no more emotive topic in medicine than suicide. In an age of evidence-based medicine in which outcomes are scrutinized, mulled over, fiercely debated, and disagreed upon, suicide stands apart. Here, there is unanimity—it is the outcome no one wanted, not even the deceased, we reason, for surely such an extreme behavior is the product of a disordered mind with judgment overcome by pain, depression, and despair."[51]

It is incumbent on clinicians not to overlook the diagnosis of depression. Evidence suggests they may do so. Data from a tertiary care MS clinic revealed that one in three people with MS had thought of attempting suicide over the course of their lives with the disease.[52] Six percent had made an attempt. A third of those who were suicidal had received no treatment, be it antidepressant medication or psychotherapy. Confirmatory evidence for these oversights come from another study which revealed that half of all MS clinic attendees with depression were either going untreated or being inadequately treated.[53] We now know that a person with MS who becomes depressed has a choice of treatments. But first, the diagnosis must be made. Failure to do so will come with consequences acutely felt.

NINE

Laughter and Tears

MY PATIENT'S PARENTS had a sense of humor. Mr. and Mrs. Jack named their first-born son Jack, and there it was on his birth certificate, little Jack Jack. It had a nice ring to it, mind you, even if it made him the butt of jokes growing up. He recalled one episode, in his late teens, when he was pulled over by a traffic cop for speeding. Asked for his name, he replied "Jack," and when the cop asked for his first name, he replied "Jack," and when the cop repeated the question and he replied "Jack" once more, the officer got irritated and, scrambling metaphors, warned that Jack was heading for "a whole bucket load of shit" if he was going to "take the piss like this." Then matters got really tense when Jack replied straight-faced that his name was Jack Jack and there was nothing anyone could do about it. A crisis was only averted when he produced his driver's license, at which point the cop, red in the face and puffed up with indignation, burst out laughing, crumpled up the ticket, commiserated with Jack and sent him on his way with another profanity and a caution.

Jack may have been able to laugh off his Jack Jack moniker, but there was nothing about his health that was amusing. Multiple sclerosis hit him early and hard, and by his late 20s he had entered a secondary progressive stage, needing a cane to get around. Despite this rapid physical deterioration, his mood remained good, and he never bemoaned his condition. Jack was blessed with a gentle, accepting temperament, and you felt good in his presence. That's right—the psychiatrist was made to feel good, buoyed by his patient's quiet and dignified demeanor, a mix of good humor, calm acceptance, and an unquenchable albeit realistic optimism about his life. With such a golden temperament, relationships came easy to him. He was happily married. He doted on his two young sons. Parents, siblings, and in-laws got along well together and were always on standby to help with tasks when needed. His friends loved him, supported him, and included him in their social plans, slowing their routines to fit in with his pace. He had much to contend with healthwise, but being bathed in this outpouring of affection made the disease seem less harsh, more manageable.

Jack came to see me three or four times a year. Watching him leave my office, dragging his feet to the accompanying click of his canes, I always wondered whether the good cheer he showed was sustained late at night, out of sight of family and friends, in those sobering moments when he was alone with his thoughts. There seemed to be no weakness in his positive attitude to life. He acknowledged he had been dealt a tough hand, no denying it. He recalled how the disease had arrived suddenly, on one of those perfect early summer days, as he lounged by his parents' swimming pool under a cloudless sky, a gentle breeze ruffling the lawn umbrella. Not a care in the world: college behind him, a good paying job, money in the bank, recently married—a happy melding of two compatible families—a baby on the way, about to move into a three-bedroom townhouse. Life was sweet. He recalls it was getting close to midday and he thought he would have another dip before lunch. Up he sprang and over he fell, the world spinning wildly around him. He tried standing again, but the ground was shifting under his feet, and down he went once more. Looking back, he considers himself lucky that he didn't fall into the pool, for he would surely have drowned. Later that evening, lying on a hospital bed in a crowded emergency room, the world still spinning like a top, he heard the words multiple sclerosis. What he remembers most of the moment, dizziness apart, was his wife's gasp and the wetness of her tears on his hand.

Seven years into his illness, Jack's condition stabilized. His disease progression, which had been relentless to that point, slowed and then seemed to stop. A year of stability followed. Walking remained a challenge, but his cognition was relatively intact apart from a slight falloff in processing speed and a verbal memory that had slipped from superior at disease onset to average over time. He still took himself off to the office every morning, driving a SUV with modified hand controls. Judging from the photographs he proudly showed me on his mobile phone at each visit, his social life had never slowed, filled as it was with a happy family and a large network of smiling, laughing, and fun-loving friends. And then, out of the blue, Jack's wife phoned, and I could immediately hear the distress in her voice. "Something is wrong with Jack," she informed me. Her calm, temperate husband, the man with a perennial smile and a kind word for everyone, could not stop crying. Nothing could turn off the tears. "The dam has finally burst," she confided. "I always wondered when my wonderful man would become depressed."

Later that week, Jack arrived for his hurriedly arranged appointment. In he hobbled, smiling his winsome smile! I smiled back. It was the Jack Jack effect. It never failed. He settled into a chair, carefully placed his walker to one side, and looked up at me, the tail end of his smile lingering as it always did, his expression conveying an infectious gaiety that was his calling card. Well, I remember thinking, how does this reconcile with his wife's anguished phone call?

In keeping with my usual practice of full disclosure whenever a relative phones to express concerns about a family member who is a patient of mine, I started off the session by letting Jack know that his wife had called me, and I told him the reason for her call. Before I could get any further, Jack's face underwent the most striking transformation. The glimmer of a smile was gone, the laugh lines around his eyes dissolved, and his attempts at speech were drowned out by a prolonged, heartbreaking sob that seemed endless. On and on it went. Jack trying vainly to gain a modicum of control over it, but just when he seemed to be on the verge of reigning it in, the emotion escaped him once more and fresh sobs erupted. As I observed this florid display of emotion, the analogy Jack's wife had used of a dam bursting seemed apt, even if her interpretation of what was driving the process was wrong. For when Jack was able to control his crying long enough to tell me how he was feeling, he strenuously denied being depressed. "I am not sad, not sad at all," he insisted over and over between racking sobs, his copious tears at odds with his protestations. I saw no reason to disbelieve him. For there, in the incongruity of Jack's responses, lay the key to diagnosis. The outward display of sadness, that flood of tears, uncontrollable at times, did not match his internal, emotional state. Jack was crying without feeling sad and, moreover, was powerless to control it. The phenomenon in which mood (subjective emotion) becomes disconnected from affect (the outward manifestation of the corresponding emotion) is the hallmark of a disorder called pseudobulbar affect. It is not limited to inappropriate crying. Uncontrollable laughter can occur, too, in the absence of happiness. The disorder is therefore defined by a paradox: tears without sadness or laughter without mirth. In some individuals, crying and laughter coexist, the one displacing the other, or merging into one another, but neither of them associated with the matching, subjective mood state. Pseudobulbar affect, also called pathological laughter and crying, affects 1 in 10 people with MS, in varying degrees of severity.[1]

The dividing line between pseudobulbar affect (PBA) and lesser degrees of emotional lability is blurred in keeping with a theme that runs through every chapter in this book: the continuum of behavioral expression. In an effort to clearly delineate PBA as a distinct phenomenon, Poeck proposed that it had to have four components: an emotional response to nonspecific stimuli, the absence of an association between affective change and the observed expression, the absence of voluntary control of facial expression, and an absence of a corresponding change in mood exceeding the period of crying or laughter.[2] This description fitted Jack Jack's presentation perfectly. To Poeck, these four criteria distinguished PBA from emotional lability, which he regarded as episodes of crying and, less frequently, laughter that were excessive but congruent to the situation in which they occurred. An example of this might be the person who cries easily during emotional scenes in a movie, or the type of individual who Frank McCourt so unforgettably described in his memoir *'Tis* as having his bladder close to his eye. (The mention of bladder recalls a frowned upon term for PBA: "emotional incontinence.") Poeck was also quite clear in excluding excessive, inappropriate crying and laughter secondary to substance abuse, psychosis, or as part of histrionic behavior from his tight definition.

Poeck was not, however, the first to describe pseudobulbar affect. That distinction fell to German neurologists Oppenheim and Siemerling more than 80 years earlier,[3] who had observed that it could occur among the signs and symptoms of pseudobulbar palsy.* The condition is found in many diverse neurological disorders, such as amyotrophic lateral sclerosis (ALS, or Lou Gehrig's disease), stroke, Alzheimer's disease, and traumatic brain injury, to give but four common examples. It arises when key neural networks that control the outward display of emotions become disrupted. These networks are widely distributed in the brain, but they all channel through a common anatomical locus, the bulbar nuclei of the brain stem. To illustrate the complexity of the processes at work, it is helpful to review each of these distinct, yet overlapping circuits individually.

In 1924, the American-born, English neurologist Kinnier Wilson published a paper in the *Journal of Neurology and Psychopathology* as part of a series entitled "Some Problems in Neurology."[4] The problem Wilson addressed was pathological laughter and crying. The mechanism that Wilson invoked to explain this disconnect of mood from affect incorporated three pivotal brain regions: the bulbar nuclei in the brain stem exerting functional control over the facial and respiratory muscles, the cortex responsible for voluntary control over the bulbar nuclei, and the connections between the bulbar nuclei and the cortex, which run in the corticospinal, corticobulbar, and corticopontine tracts. Damage

---

* The "pseudo" descriptor refers to the presence of bulbar signs, such as dysarthria (difficulty with speech) and dysphagia (difficulty with swallowing), in the absence of a bulbar (brainstem) lesion. The symptoms arise from an upper motor neuron lesion entailing bilateral disturbance of the corticobulbar tracts that exert supranuclear control over the brain stem, bulbar nuclei.

to one or more of these regions could in theory disconnect the bulbar nuclei from higher cortical control, in the process triggering uncontrollable laughter or crying divorced from a matching mood. Almost 100 years later, the skeleton of the network postulated by Wilson is still relevant, except now we know that the neural circuitry involved is more intricate.[5,6]

Let us start with a pathway that underlies conscious emotion. To illustrate what conscious emotion is, I would like you to answer the following questions: What are the birthdates of your children, or spouse, or parents? What is the date of your wedding anniversary? To answer these questions, you have to make an effort consciously by accessing memories that are stored in the hippocampus. As noted previously in Chapter 4, the hippocampus is important in consolidating memories from short-term to long-term, and damage to this region can result in significant memory impairment. Being able to recall personally important dates like birthdays and anniversaries demands a conscious effort on the part of the person accessing the memories. This process also comes with emotional overtones. For example, if you are happily married and still in love with your partner, then the recall of an anniversary should be associated with a matched emotion—happiness. The same holds true for memories of your children's birthdays. These are enjoyable events, a time of celebration, and an opportunity to express love and affection. Consciously recalling an anniversary dinner in a lovely restaurant, or the romantic anniversary getaway to an island resort, or the low-key fun dinner at the greasy spoon just up the road where you held hands and reminisced about your wedding day all those years ago, places demands on your memory. You have to summon up these memories, which once accessed invoke a feeling of happiness paired with the event. Conversely, if you have gone through a bitter divorce associated with a difficult period of feeling sadness, anger, regret, and despair, then the memory of what should have been a happy time has become tainted and replaced by a slew of negative feelings. Either way, the brain network that invests these memories with emotions entails connections between the hippocampus and the cingulate cortex. Reciprocal connections are present to the dorsolateral prefrontal cortex, a region involved in working memory and integral to processing information and assigning conscious awareness.

Contrast this with unconscious or involuntary emotions. This feeling is visceral, instinctive. It arises involuntarily in response to an external event or the memory of that event. The emotion may be pleasant or unpleasant, depending on the event. For example, you are traveling in a car. You turn the corner and there it is, fresh road kill, right in front of you, a grisly spectacle of macerated flesh and fur, intestines like uncooked sausages strewn across the road, bright red smudges of blood glistening in the morning sunshine. Your first response is to recoil, grimace, and avert your gaze. The sight is nauseating, and your accompanying emotions are unpleasant, a mix of disgust and horror. The whole episode, from first sighting to gaze averted is no more than a second or two, time enough for you to be flooded by waves of strong emotions, which linger even as you accelerate away from the carnage.

The same mechanism driving this visceral emotion is in action when it comes to pleasanter feelings. Imagine sleeping through your morning alarm clock and once awake having to rush to work, forsaking your breakfast apart from a quick espresso. Your day at the office is full, and in keeping with your poor start to the day, things unfold somewhat haphazardly, ensuring there is little time for lunch, which is reduced to a tired salad that you leave half uneaten. By the time you get home in the evening you are famished. You walk in through the front door and your senses are assailed by the most heavenly aromas. Your partner, who enjoys cooking, has experimented with a new recipe, and the smells emanating from the kitchen have you salivating. The meal is ready, timed to perfection, and as you hurriedly wash your hands, your thoughts are pleasantly occupied by food. The emotions that accompany your keen anticipation of what is to come are those of happiness and joy, the antithesis of what you felt when you rounded the corner and came across the road kill recently. The pleasant smell of food expertly cooked entices you, attracts you, pulls you toward the dining room, which you enter with a smile and a heart full of affection for the person who has gone to all this effort of creating such a lovely moment. These emotions also arise without thought or effort, triggered involuntarily by the power of smell.

The emotive pull of scent is powerfully revealed in the duty-free shops that await the traveler emerging from the security check points at international airports. Shelves laden with bottles of perfume. Row upon row of multicolored, exotically shaped bottles, many displaying the names of the world's great fashion houses and designers, all united in a single purpose—to entice you into buying them by seducing you with smell. A huge, expensive industry has flourished for centuries by gaining access to your heart through your nose. The functional neuroanatomy of smell and emotion intersect seamlessly, the connections immediate, visceral, unconscious. And such is the power of the neural network, should the emotions generated be pleasing, arousing, or seductive, then the journey from sniff to open wallet is all but assured.

The key anatomical regions that control the generation of unconscious emotions, such as fear, disgust, and the happiness associated with pleasure, include the amygdala and orbitofrontal cortex. These regions process information from the cortical association areas and modulate visceral and motor responses to this information through connections to the brainstem, basal ganglia, and hypothalamus. Of note is that the first cranial nerve, the olfactory nerve, runs from the nose up through the cribriform plate of the skull to synapse in the orbitofrontal cortex, which helps explain the emotive power of smell. While the neural connections that link the orbitofrontal cortex with the amygdala are distinct from those that underpin the conscious emotion circuitry with hubs in the hippocampus and anterior cingulate, the two circuits are in contact through the infracallosal cingulate.

There is a third neural circuit that plays an important role in controlling the outward display of emotion, or affect. Social etiquette is an important factor that modulates our emotional responses to external events. The humor of a comedian and the silly antics of children elicit laughter. Funerals and memorial services demand a different display of emotion, the sadness of the occasion dictating a somber expression as a sign of respect to those in mourning. Not all situations are so clearcut, however. The person who slips on an oily patch may look ridiculous in doing so, the flailing arms and legs unable to prevent a funny-looking pratfall, but whatever smiles are triggered by this mishap quickly evaporate when we realize the unfortunate person has been hurt in the process. The smile or laughter is quickly stifled, to be replaced by a concerned expression reflecting the sympathy that the circumstances require. These socially mediated nuances of affect are learned responses, culturally mediated to a degree. Like all behavioral responses, they are controlled by neural pathways, and here the relevant brain network includes the cerebellum with connections to the prefrontal cortex. With disruption of this circuit, the individual may receive incomplete information that fails to imbue an external event with the correct social and cognitive context. The result is a display of emotion that is inappropriate or excessive.

This overview of the functional neuroanatomy of PBA reveals the many widely dispersed brain regions potentially implicated in the syndrome, including the brain stem, cerebellum, hippocampus, anterior cingulate, orbitofrontal and dorsolateral prefrontal cortices, the sensory association areas, and the motor cortex. While the networks funnel into a single final relay station in the bulbar nuclei of the brain stem, PBA can arise from lesions far removed from the brain stem, a phenomenon that accounts for the "pseudo" component to the syndrome's name.

With this in mind, one can now appreciate how a disease like MS, with widespread cortical and white matter involvement, can disconnect pivotal circuits at multiple points. MRI provides confirmatory evidence of this, in particular an association with bilateral lesions, suggesting that in some individuals it might take disruption of networks in both hemispheres before the affect becomes dysregulated. In an MRI study of people with MS comparing those with and without PBA, the former were found to have a significantly greater lesion volume in bilateral parietal and orbitofrontal, left medial superior frontal, and brain stem regions. The lesions, both hypo- and hyperintense, could account for close to 80% of the variance in explaining the presence of PBA, indicating that uncontrollable laughter and crying is essentially the product of brain changes.[7] If we think back to Chapter 8, this is almost double the variance associated with MRI-demonstrable brain changes in depressed people with MS. This difference underscores the more complex etiology of depression, where psychosocial factors, as we have seen, hold greater sway.

The presence of a significant brain lesion load in people with PBA suggests the presence of comorbid cognitive problems too. Three MS studies confirm as much. In the first, 152 people with MS attending a hospital-based clinic were screened by researchers in my lab for PBA with the Pathological Laugher and Crying Scale (PLACS).[1] Fifteen individuals were found to have the disorder, of whom 11 agreed to undergo further, limited neuropsychological testing. This group comprised six people with pathological crying, three with uncontrollable laugher, and two with mixed crying and laughing. The majority had entered a progressive disease course, reflected in a group Expanded Disability Status Scale (EDSS) score of 6.4, which is indicative of someone requiring constant bilateral assistance with canes, crutches, or both to walk. When the cognitive results were compared to those from 13 people with MS but no PBA (matched for sex, age, level of education, EDSS, duration of MS, and disease course), the PBA group was found to have a lower performance IQ and greater impairment on three subscales of the Wechsler Adult Intelligence Scale–Revised[8] (arithmetic, digit-symbol, and picture arrangement). Moreover, a closer look at the digit-span results revealed more prominent deficits on the Digits Backward, but not the Digits Forward component. Taken collectively, these cognitive results indicated further compromise in processing speed and working memory in people with MS and PBA.

In a second study from the same group of people with and without PBA, my lab reported the results from three tests that probe executive function: the Stroop, Wisconsin Card Sorting Test (WCST), and Controlled Oral Word Association Test (COWAT).[9] The first two tests will be familiar to readers from the earlier chapter on executive function. The COWAT probes verbal fluency as an index of executive function, with the person being tested required to name as many words as possible beginning with the letters F, A, and S and given one minute for each letter. Once more, greater deficits were present in the PBA group on the Stroop and COWAT with a trend in the same direction for the WCST.

The final cognitive study entailed a retrospective chart review of 153 people with MS who had attended an MS outpatient clinic.[10] All had been administered a battery of cognitive tests and self-report scales designed to detect PBA with the seven-item self-administered Center for Neurologic Study–Lability Scale (CNS-LS)[11] and ascertain symptoms of depression and anxiety with the Hospital Anxiety and Depression Scale.[12] The results overlapped to a degree with those reported earlier; namely, an association between the presence of PBA and deficits in executive function and verbal learning.

The phenomenological differences between PBA and depression also extend to treating the two conditions, although even here, there are certain similarities as well. While depression can respond well to psychotherapy, this intervention is ineffective in a condition like PBA, which is neurologically hardwired and, as such, etiologically relatively independent of psychological factors. To be sure, talk therapy can be supportive and can potentially limit the distress that comes with PBA, but it cannot halt the uncontrollable laughter and crying. Antidepressant medication, on the other hand, can. The earliest evidence of this emerged in 1985 in a double-blind crossover study of 12 people with MS and PBA, which showed that amitriptyline, a tricyclic antidepressant drug that dates from 1960, significantly reduced symptoms compared to placebo.[13] Furthermore, improvement occurred with modest doses. Subsequent open-label trials and case studies confirmed the benefits of antidepressant medication, albeit with the serotonin reuptake inhibitor drug fluoxetine[14] and the anticonvulsant and mood stabilizer valproic acid.[15]

The challenge of treating PBA with antidepressant medications is twofold—namely, tolerating side effects and a reluctance on the part of people to take psychotropic medications in general. With respect to the former, a dry mouth, constipation, and most significantly, sexual dysfunction can make compliance with treatment patchy at best, thereby diluting the benefits of treatment. It is not unusual to have people with PBA find themselves in the uncomfortable position of having to choose between better control of their laughter and crying versus the frustration and embarrassment of sexual dysfunction. Here, it is important to view this ambivalence in the context of a disease that has an onset in young and middle-aged people—that demographic which is sexually the most active. Add a drug that takes away yet one more important function, and the resistance to drug compliance is not hard to understand.

These challenges with prescribing antidepressant medications open the door to a new, different class of medication for PBA. AVP-923 is a compound containing dextromethorphan (DM) and quinidine (Q), the latter inhibiting the rapid first pass metabolism of the former. DM alone was first trialed as a neuroprotective agent in people with ALS given its anti-glutamate properties, but the results were poor, perhaps because of the rapid, extensive metabolism of the drug. However, coadministration of quinidine at doses below that used to treat cardiac arrhythmias essentially overrides the metabolism of DM. While combined DM and Q did not prove a game changer for people with ALS, a serendipitous finding was that the drug inhibited pathological laughter and crying, which occurs in a third[16] to a half[17] of people with ALS. This led to a 28-day randomized, double-blind trial of DM+Q (30 mg of each) given twice daily versus DM or Q alone in people with ALS. PBA was measured with the CNS-LS. The combination therapy was found to be significantly more effective than either component alone. Of note is that a reduction in PBA was associated with a significant increase in measures of quality of life and quality of relationships.[18]

The *Oxford English Dictionary* defines serendipity as "the faculty of making happy and unexpected discoveries by accident, or when looking for something else," and *Merriam-Webster's Collegiate Dictionary* defines it as "the faculty or phenomenon of finding valuable or agreeable things not sought for." *Serendip* (or *Serendib*) is the old Arabic name for Ceylon, now called Sri Lanka. The origin of the word "serendipity" may be traced to an old Persian fairy tale, *The Three Princes of Serendip*, in which the heroes in their travels unwittingly stumbled across new discoveries and sources of wisdom. The word has a long and distinguished history in drug discovery.[19] What is particularly notable is the reach of serendipity into drugs that modify thoughts, emotions, and behavior. Nine of the 11 drugs mentioned in Thomas Ban's erudite paper "The Role of Serendipity in Drug Research"[19] are psychotropic agents.

They include the sedatives potassium bromide and choral hydrate, the mood stabilizer lithium, the hallucinogen lysergic acid (or LSD), the anxiolytics meprobamate and chlordiazepoxide, the antipsychotic chlorpromazine, and two antidepressants, the tricyclic imipramine and the monoamine oxidase inhibitor iproniazid. The only two nonpsychotropic drugs that make Ban's list have both, in very different ways, transformed health care—penicillin and sildenafil, the latter better known by its trade name, Viagra. To this list, one may now add the only treatment for PBA that is approved by the US Food and Drug Administration (FDA), a drug that can turn off the laughter and crying of PBA, another notable psychotropic: the combination of dextromethorphan and quinidine known by the trade name Nuedexta.

The first clinical trial of DM+Q in people with MS and PBA was a 12-week, randomized, double-blind, placebo-controlled study in which the dosage, as in the ALS study, remained at 30 mg for each component.[20] Major depression was an exclusion criterion. Significant improvements were seen in the treatment group—namely, a 7.7-point decline in CNS-LS scores (versus 3.3 in the placebo group) and a falloff in weekly PBA episodes from 14.1 to 4.7 (versus 17.3 to 11.5 in the placebo group).

Concerns over cardiac toxicity linked to high-dose quinidine led to a third well-powered DM+Q study that included people with MS and ALS. This 12-week, randomized, double-blind, placebo-controlled, Safety, Tolerability, and Efficacy Results (STAR) study compared the efficacy and side effects of DM+Q (30/10 mg), DM+Q (20/10 mg), and placebo.[21] Once more, people with severe depression were excluded. The primary outcome measure was a reduction in the PBA-episode daily rate, which fell by almost 50% in both active treatment groups. A remission in PBA, which was defined by no episodes in the previous two weeks of the study, was reached by 47.3% in the DM+Q (30/10mg) group, 51.4% in the DM+Q (20/10mg) group, and 2.4% in the placebo group. Dizziness and diarrhea emerged as side effects that were statistically more frequent in both active groups compared to the placebo one. The STAR trial determined that the optimum dextromethorphan-quinidine dosage ratio was 20/10 mg and was pivotal in getting FDA approval for the drug. Potential participants with cardiac disease were excluded from the STAR trial, and the drug still comes with a warning that it should not be taken by someone with cardiac disease.

There is a happy clinical coda to this chapter. Jack Jack's pseudobulbar affect resolved completely with treatment. After two years of no PBA episodes, he asked if he could discontinue the drug. He phased out treatment over the course of a month and then held his breath waiting for symptoms to return. They never did. Soon thereafter, his MS stabilized in response to beginning a trial of siponimod, a disease-modifying therapy approved for use in people with secondary progressive disease.[22] On the 20th anniversary of his first appointment with me (he remembered the date, I did not), Jack returned bringing his wife and two children, lovely young adults with that same open expression and twinkle in the eye that distinguished their father. Clearly the right genes had been passed on, and as I sat there observing and marveling at this happy, loving family, I quietly hoped that other more ominous genes that had tried and failed to bring down their father would bypass the next, delightful generation of Jacks.

TEN

A Break with Reality

THE NEUROLOGIST'S SHORT, cryptic referral note told me very little. "A 50-year-old man with a year of odd behavior that is out of keeping with this usual personality. MS appears stable. A couple of new lesions on his MRI. If you could see him soon, that would be appreciated by me and, I suspect, his family."

Two weeks later, the man who showed up for his appointment clearly did not want to be here. Eduardo entered my office hesitantly, looking over his shoulder as he did so. In a pattern of behavior that would become familiar to me in the months to come, he slowly scanned the room with a hypervigilant gaze, completed a 360-degree sweep, crossed his arms defiantly over a bulky jacket, and furtively made eye contact. My introduction was met with silence.

Rather than jump right into the reason for the consultation, I tried to lessen the tension by making a little small talk. This was greeted with a look of deep mistrust and more awkward silence. With the clock ticking and a long list of patients still to be seen, I did not have the option afforded psychoanalysts of letting the silence speak for itself and interpreting it accordingly. Instead, I reverted to my usual, more focused, approach and let Eduardo know that he had been referred by his neurologist, and that I would like to take his history and thereafter perhaps be in a position to make some recommendations, if need be.

What emerged, haltingly, grudgingly over the next 50 minutes was a litany of complaints that spoke to an entrenched set of persecutory beliefs that had led to the loss of a job, friendships, and a marriage. All that remained of his once large and vibrant social circle were two teenage children, and even they were drifting from him. I asked him how he could account for this. And with that question, the floodgates opened.

Eduardo was an economist. He had obtained his PhD from the University of Lima, Peru. His area of expertise was game theory, as applied to emerging markets in postcolonial societies. His work had been widely cited internationally, and for a few years he had held a position at the World Bank. When President Alberto Fujimori declared a state of emergency and suspended the Peruvian constitution in the early 1990s, Eduardo left Peru on a one-way ticket and, using connections forged over the years with Canadian colleagues, found a home in Ottawa, Ontario, and a job in the Canadian federal government. Within a year, he was able to call for his wife and two young children to join him. Despite the upheaval of enforced immigration, the family prospered. Fifteen good years followed.

Then things started to go wrong. His voice rising in anger, Eduardo divulged that jealous colleagues began conspiring against him. They stole his ideas. They spoke of him behind his back. They shunned him in the cafeteria. They stopped inviting him for an after-work drink. Promotions were denied. He was sure his phone had been tapped. He was convinced that his car had been scratched on purpose. He was certain that contacts had been established between the Canadian and Peruvian governments with the aim of having him returned to his country of birth. Worst of all, his wife did not believe him when he complained to her of his persecution. She told him he was imaging things. She scolded him for upsetting their children with his tales of plots and the conniving behavior of politicians. It was incredible that such things could be happening here, in Canada—a country that had taken him in only to spit him out again.

Paranoia is, of course, not unusual to come across in a psychiatric practice. What made Eduardo's history notable from a neuropsychiatric perspective, however, was the part that he omitted. Two years before the onset of his delusional thinking, he lost sensation in his left foot. It returned after a few months but was followed by blurry vision in his right eye, which never completed resolved. Then the sensory loss returned, but this time it was from the waist down and accompanied by difficulties with bladder and bowel. The diagnosis of multiple sclerosis was confirmed, and a disease-modifying drug was started, seemingly to good effect. Symptoms improved considerably and in time faded into the background, where Eduardo regarded them with a mild annoyance. Rather, his attention was increasingly consumed by what he was convinced were the evolving plots against him and the concerted efforts of a state-sponsored system to bring him down. He filed a grievance against his employers, which had the unfortunate effect of further alienating his colleagues, thereby providing additional fuel for his paranoia. By the time he came to see me, his life had unraveled.

The hallmark of psychosis is a disturbance in reality testing associated with absent or poor insight. Eduardo's beliefs, unrelated to mood, were clearly false, and yet he held tenaciously to them. The etiological question that needed addressing was whether his disturbed mental state was a consequence of his multiple sclerosis or a chance occurrence. He also needed treatment.

Psychosis, broadly defined as the presence of delusions and/or hallucinations in the absence of delirium, is not a formal psychiatric diagnosis. Rather, it is a descriptive term that captures the phenomenology of what happens when a person loses touch with reality and when delusions (defined as fixed, false beliefs held despite evidence to the contrary and not culturally sanctioned) and hallucinations (defined as perceptions in the absence of external stimuli) occur. There are a number of psychiatric disorders in which psychosis appears. Using the nomenclature of the fifth edition of the American Psychiatric Association's *Diagnostic and Statistical Manual of Mental Disorders* (*DSM-5*)[1] there are disorders in which psychosis is integral to the condition, a core clinical feature, without which the diagnoses cannot be made. Examples here include schizophrenia, schizoaffective disorder, delusional disorder, and brief psychotic disorder. Then there are conditions in which psychosis may be found occasionally, such as substance-related and addictive disorders (e.g., involving cannabis, phencyclidine, or amphetamines) and mood disorders (e.g., major depression and bipolar affective disorder).

It is estimated that the lifetime prevalence of psychosis is around 1%. Put another way, one person in 100 in the general population will lose touch with reality (i.e., become psychotic) over the course of his or her lifetime. Multiple sclerosis is common in certain regions, too, with a lifetime prevalence of 0.1% to 0.01% (the variability accounted for by latitude). The possibility of the two disorders arising in the same person for unrelated reasons is therefore 0.5 to 1 per 100,000 people. Any increase in this number suggests a causal link, and this has been explored in two epidemiological studies. Given universal health care coverage in Canada, all individuals seen by physicians are given diagnoses, which are coded according to the International Classification of Diseases (ninth edition).[2] Data from the province of Alberta between 1994 and 2003 revealed that 10,367 out of 2.45 million residents over the age of 15 years had MS, giving an estimated prevalence of 330 per 100,000 people, in keeping historically with Alberta's high prevalence rate.[3] Psychotic illness was also coded and was divided into two categories: nonorganic (schizophrenia-spectrum disorders, delusional disorders, and other nonorganic psychoses) and organic (which included drug-induced psychoses, transient organic psychoses, and other organic psychotic disorders). The central message that emerged from this semantic and taxonomic minefield was that psychosis was found to occur in 2% to 3% of people with MS, a significant increase relative to those in the general population without MS. The rates were particularly elevated in younger people with MS; namely, in the 15-to-24-year-old age group. This age differential is not surprising given that the average age of onset of psychosis in the general population is the late teens and early 20s, a developmental period of heightened vulnerability.

A subsequent Canadian study[4] with a broader reach (British Columbia, Nova Scotia, Manitoba, and Quebec) and a tighter diagnostic focus (schizophrenia) confirmed a higher incidence—that is, the rate of oc-currence of new cases. Adjusting for year and sex, the age-standardized incidence was 74% higher in the MS group compared to the matched general population. The incidence was lower in women than in men, which does not fit with the general psychiatry data and declined slightly over time. When it came to prevalence—that is, the proportion of cases in the population at a given period of time—the age-adjusted rate was again higher in the MS group compared to the matched general popu-lation group, but this fell short of statistical significance. Unlike with depression, anxiety, and bipolar affective disorder, the prevalence was lower in women than men.

The Canadian epidemiological data provide compelling evidence that people with MS are more vulnerable to developing a psychotic illness. However, the same conclusion was not reached in a systematic review that cast a wider geographical net.[5] The challenge here was compounded by diagnostic inconsistency—some studies referred to psychosis, others to schizophrenia, and one to brief psychotic disorders—and differences in control and comparator groups. As a result, the findings were incon-sistent and suggested that further study was required.

What is notable about the MS-psychosis literature is the absence of a prospective study. This indicates that the actual number of people with MS who become psychotic is very small, notwithstanding the epidemi-ological data pointing toward an elevated risk. The literature, however, is replete with case reports. A systematic review of these case reports identified 91 cases with diverse diagnoses encompassing primary psy-chotic disorders and mood disorders associated with psychotic features.[6] Unlike in the population-based studies of MS-related psychosis, there was a preponderance of women. The mean sample age of 34.4 years, while still young by MS standards, is relatively old by the yardstick of psychosis onset within the general population. Of particular interest was the observation that at least 26 people had been treated with steroids in the acute phase of their psychosis, for the most part to good effect, sug-gesting that the psychotic episode was deemed integral to their under-lying neurological disease and akin, in theory, to an MS relapse. This point fits with a number of case reports documenting psychosis as the first presenting feature of multiple sclerosis.[7-9]

In the absence of prospective studies, informative retrospective case series fill the void. One such report identified 15 people (nine were men) with MS and psychosis assessed and treated over a five-year period at a tertiary care center.[10] The mean age of onset of psychosis was 39 years, and the majority of individuals had a progressive form of MS. A breakdown of psychotic signs and symptoms revealed the following, in order of frequency: persecutory delusions (87%), lack of insight (80%), delusions of reference (53%; this refers to an individual misinterpreting innocuous or coincidental events as having some personal, usually negative, significance), auditory hallucinations (43%), grandiose delusions (27%), delusions of passivity (27%; a belief that one is being controlled by some external force), visual hallucinations (20%), somatic hallucinations (20%), and thought alienation (20%; a belief that one's thoughts are being inserted, withdrawn, or broadcast).

When it comes to causation in individual cases, various possibilities need to be considered. Epidemiological data may make the case for an elevated rate of psychosis in MS in general, but the clinician, faced with a person with MS who has lost touch with reality, cannot automatically attribute the person's delusions or hallucinations to MS. In this instance, the temporal sequence of events can prove helpful. A causal link is most unlikely when the onset of psychosis precedes the diagnosis of MS by many years. When this occurs, and psychosis began in the late teens or early 20s, the likelihood of the two disorders occurring by chance is high. However, when psychosis arises in close proximity to the onset of MS, or should MS begin well before the mental illness, then the possibility of a causal link must be considered. In these instances, brain imaging can offer some help.

During my PhD studies in Professor Maria Ron's lab at the Institute of Neurology, Queen Square in London, we compared MRI data between a group of people with (n=10) and without (n=10) psychosis individually matched for age, disability, duration of MS, and disease type.[11] Significant imaging differences were found, with the psychotic group having a higher lesion score in the left temporal horn and trigone area. While these regions overlap with those identified in the schizophrenia literature, both at postmortem[12] and on MRI,[13] it is also true that many people with MS who have similarly distributed lesions do not become psychotic. What the imaging results, therefore, more plausibly suggest is that lesions in regions implicated in psychosis—namely, the medial temporal lobes—take on added significance in people with MS who have a pre-MS vulnerability to the development of psychosis. This susceptibility lies along a continuum with numerous risk and protective factors (familial, environmental, and psychosocial) proposed for psychosis in general.[14] In the person with MS with one or more of these putative factors, the presence of lesions in an anatomically key region may therefore be the precipitant that tips the scales toward psychosis. The same interpretation is applicable to the imaging data available in 50 of the 91 cases that made it into a systematic review of psychosis in people with MS.[6] Almost two-thirds of these individuals had predominantly frontotemporal lesions. Contrast enhancing lesions indicative of active disease were also common.

Before leaving the question of causality, the potential role played by medication in psychosis deserves mention. Despite isolated case reports linking psychosis to treatment of MS with interferon β-1b[15] and interferon β-1a,[16] there is no compelling overall evidence that disease-modifying therapies are the culprit. Steroids, however, are of more interest, as they have been linked to an array of behavioral effects—including psychosis—in the general psychiatry,[17,18] neuropsychiatry,[19] neurology,[20] and multiple sclerosis[21] literature. At the same time, steroids have been used, often successfully, to treat psychotic episodes associated with a flare in MS.[6] This seeming contradiction may be accounted for by a couple of explanations. The first is that in the context of florid psychosis triggered by an MS exacerbation, the powerful anti-inflammatory benefits of a steroid hold sway. The second possibility entails a more nuanced looked at the neurology/MS-steroid-side-effect literature. In a general neurology context, steroid use is most closely associated with mania, not psychosis.[20] A manic patient may become psychotic, but the important point is that, should psychosis ensue, this change is usually mood related. This finding meshes with an earlier observation that people with MS who become hypomanic or manic on steroid treatment are more likely to have a history of depression preceding use or a family history of depression and/or alcoholism.[22] Furthermore, there is evidence that steroid treatment should not necessarily be discontinued in the person with MS who has become manic. Rather, the introduction of lithium, a mood stabilizing agent, may allow for completion of a full course of steroid treatment, with attendant benefits.[23] Thus, we return yet again to the continuum of risk.

How, then, should the person with MS and psychosis be treated? In the rare case of psychosis precipitated by treatment with a disease-modifying therapy, the drug should be stopped. As noted earlier, should the clinician have evidence from the neurological examination and MRI, ideally with contrast enhancement, that the delusions or hallucinations are likely part of an MS relapse, then steroids can be tried. There is, however, no MS-related clinical trial to provide guidance here, but case reports show that steroids alone may not be sufficient.[6] If that is the case, antipsychotic medication will be needed. Finally, for those individuals whose psychosis is not relapse related, antipsychotic treatment is the mainstay of therapy. Once more, there is no randomized controlled MS trial to point the way. Isolated case reports and retrospective case histories support the use of the newer, atypical antipsychotic agents, such as olanzapine, quetiapine, aripiprazole, and risperidone,[10,24] the latter drug also given in depot (long-acting intramuscular) form.[25] The outcome is perhaps a little better than it is in a primary psychotic illness. In one-third of individuals whose psychosis was not considered part of an MS exacerbation, full recovery occurred after six months of antipsychotic treatment.[10]

Before concluding, let us return to Eduardo and his troubled life. The age of onset of his psychosis was much later than one sees in a primary psychiatric illness. It also postdated his neurological disorder by at least two years. His MRI spoke of active disease, although he was not currently experiencing a relapse. These three facts weighted the argument in favor of MS as the causative factor in his psychosis. Armed with this theoretical evidence, I broached the subject of treatment with him. Eduardo was having none of it. Why should he take antipsychotic treatment, he demanded to know, when the problem lay with others? Dropping his voice to a conspiratorial whisper, he edged closer to me and, with the back of his hand shielding his mouth, divulged, "It's them, not me," which he repeated for emphasis.

In that one pithy summation of how Eduardo viewed his predicament lay the challenge of treating his paranoia. I certainly tried, but the absence of insight presented an insuperable barrier. No matter how I approached the subject of medication, I was rebuffed. His defense was watertight, his resolve steely, and his argument unwavering. He had no difficulty accepting the diagnosis of multiple sclerosis and taking his daily glatiramer acetate injections, but when it came to a discussion of antipsychotic medication, it was like flipping a light switch. Logic instantaneously evaporated revealing a fixation with the government and his conviction that a diabolical plot had been hatched to bring him down. The belief was so well-encapsulated that if one steered the conversation into different territory, his discourse was rational, lucid, learned, and devoid of the hostility and animus that were attached like barnacles to his persecutory delusions. I saw repeated evidence of this. In order to try to build a trusting relationship with him, I recall once asking him about his PhD, and what followed was a lengthy, erudite, and passionate account of the work that had opened doors to an international career. Eduardo seemed to enjoy these types of conversations, and it was clear to me that he was lonely, his paranoia having cut him off from friends, colleagues, and increasingly, his family too. He readily admitted to being socially isolated, but he saw this as one more malignant design on the part of his persecutors. It was not enough that they had destroyed his career—they were also working to destroy his entire life. That's how despicable they were.

A couple of months after we first met, I received a call from Eduardo's wife. By now, the couple was living apart and the children were with her. Eduardo must have told her of his appointments with me and she wanted one too. I mentioned the call to Eduardo, and he agreed to have her come along with him. I never expected her to arrive with the children and neither did Eduardo, but he seemed pleased to see them. His daughters, on the other hand, appeared wary and apprehensive, their embraces perfunctory, their smiles forced. The session started off calmly enough, but about 10 minutes into it, his wife let slip the word "crazy." Mayhem ensued. Like a flash, Eduardo jumped on the word, demanding to know what she meant by it, and before she could answer, he began fulminating against her and the Peruvian and Canadian governments. He was livid, shouting, the spittle flying as the words gushed forth, one persecutory belief merging with another, a torrent of pent-up fury and frustration that swatted aside his wife's tearful apology and the pitiful pleas of his children for papa to calm down. Oblivious to his family's distress, Eduardo continued his rant. My attempts to calm him failed too. He looked right through me as he tore into his imaginary tormenters. He had the floor to himself now and was not going to yield it until he could spend every last drop of accumulated hurt and humiliation, years' worth of "shit that I have had to swallow." He couldn't even put the brakes on when his wife stood up and, beckoning the children to follow her, backed out my office, mouthing a silent apology to me and conveying in look and gesture her utter despair.

When at last Eduardo's rage abated, he lapsed into sullen silence. There was no remorse for his explosive behavior, no regret for terrifying his children or reducing his wife to tears. His lack of empathy was chilling. He saw himself as the aggrieved party, the feelings of his family inconsequential compared to the pain he had been forced to endure. On one level, he could see that his family was broken, but he reasoned that the distress that came with this was his alone. An inability to see beyond the margins of his own distorted beliefs prevented him from appreciating his family's pain even though he claimed to love them still. "But how can they love me," he asked rhetorically, "if they also consider me crazy?" All of which revealed to him with crystal clarity that his love was now one-sided.

After six months of futile endeavor on my part, Eduardo decided to end contact. I could not enforce treatment for, notwithstanding his major mental illness, he never met one of the three criteria necessary for certification. He had never been suicidal. Despite his anger at his family, there had never been any homicidal intent. Rather, he never stopped professing his love for a family who had "kicked him in the balls." And he could look after himself, even if he now appeared shabby and unkempt, his appearance far removed from his dapper World Bank days. At his last appointment, Eduardo's aloofness and hostility seemed to weaken momentarily. He was halfway out the door when he paused, as though collecting himself, and turned slowly to stare at me. "You know, Doc, you're a nice guy," he told me, almost sympathetically, "but you just never got it." A look of ineffable sadness passed over his features. "You see, it's them, not me! Always has been." The cri de coeur of a paranoid man. And then he was gone.

ELEVEN

The Paradox of Time and Space

Redux

THE YEAR WAS 1945 when Churchill imparted his "command the moment to remain" wisdom to the two junior officers assigned to his security detail. He could not have known that his advice, the distillation of all his long, varied, and at times tumultuous experiences, would 30 years later become one of the central guiding principles of mindfulness-based therapy as first described by Jon Kabat-Zinn.[1] Kabat-Zinn did not, of course, have Churchill in mind when he was formulating his influential theory, but instead he was drawing on Buddhist philosophy and teachings going back thousands of years. It is also highly unlikely that Churchill was thinking of the Buddha as he looked over the serene waters of Lake Como, for there is no evidence he ever felt a calling for Eastern philosophies. Great minds intersect in unforeseeable ways.

As we have seen in the chapters on depression, psychotherapy can lift mood, improve MRI markers of disease activity, and boost the immune system. It can also help counteract the twin challenges of constricted space and slowed time that accompany increasing disability. As this book draws to a close, here is a final case history, which makes this point.

Ryan was 22 years of age when he was diagnosed with multiple sclerosis. Four years earlier, fresh out of high school, he had moved into a small apartment after landing a job at a hardware megastore with long aisles of goods stacked high to the ceiling. It was physically demanding work, what with all the walking and climbing up ladders that ran on railings along the aisles. Limb weakness slowed him at first, but he plowed on. Ten years into his illness, the work was beyond him. He was a popular employee, and the company found him another position, tracking inventory. Now he sat in a small, airless basement room in front of a computer keeping tabs on the goods that flowed in and out of the store. Fatigue and boredom were his twin challenges. His boss would catch him napping at his desk and bawl him out for being lazy. When the economy tanked with the subprime mortgage crisis, the company restructured and Ryan was out of a job.

Anxieties over finding work were compounded by challenges that now complicated his friendships. Friday night was typically spent with friends at a local bar. One hot, humid evening, Ryan's neurogenic bladder conspired with an inaccessible bathroom and he wet himself. Amidst howls and hoots of laughter, Ryan sheepishly made his way home to clean himself before collapsing into bed and sleeping 14 hours straight. This debacle changed how he socialized. To be sure, he still dragged himself to the bar at the end of the week, but now he nursed one beer for the evening, a change that perplexed his drinking buddies, who reacted with amusement at first but then with increasing irritation as the night wore on. The pressure to keep up with the pace of drinking was hard to resist, and the more he said no, the more he seemed to become marginalized from the group revelry. Sobriety was seen as an affront, a rebuke to socially engrained behavior that had for years defined the parameters of their end-of-week get-together. To have a buddy in their midst who remained sober and, yes, somber too, undercut the party spirit and was mistakenly seen as a rebuke to the time-honored tradition of washing away a week of toil by getting hammered. Not one of his friends ever made the connection between his limp and his incontinence. No one ever asked him why he seemed so quiet and withdrawn. All they saw was someone who was no longer one of them, who seemed different, removed, not a whole lot of fun. It only took a couple of months or so for Ryan to feel an outsider, excluded. What had once been something to look forward to now became an added stress. He cut an increasingly forlorn and distant figure, unconsciously sidelined by a group of young men in robust health who wanted no early reminders of the infirmities that could come with age and illness.

Finding a new job became futile. The process of rejection came to feel scripted. The charade, which is how he viewed it, invariably played out like this: The worrying signs appeared early in the interview. He saw it immediately on the faces of those interviewing him. No sooner had he darkened their doorway than he observed the beginnings of a smile morph into alarm, surprise, and at times even horror. As he shuffled forward with his cane, there were panicked attempts to get smiles back in place, except it could never be done convincingly, and the result was a mishmash of competing emotions, the rictus of forced joviality compounding the awkward start. Once Ryan settled in a chair, there began the steady downward drift of formulaic questions and well-rehearsed answers. The process kept going long enough so as not to cause any of the parties further embarrassment, and then it was over, the phony handshakes and eyes awkwardly diverted, the stock phrase "we'll be in touch with our decision" ringing hollow because everyone in that room knew what the outcome would be. Many years of hard work had been enough to earn a decent reference, but Ryan could never shake the impression that if one read between the lines of his testimonial, what seeped out was pity. He thought of asking his employer for a different reference, one that omitted well-meaning but ham-handed references to "courage," "adversity," and "climbing the steepest mountain." But then he thought better of it. After all, everything was starkly revealed the moment his interviewers clapped eyes on him, their job ads trumpeting "equal opportunity employer" no more than a sop to human rights watchdogs.

The failure to find work meant no money was coming in, and a disability allowance could not cover expenses. As Ryan began slipping into debt, the only solution was to move back in with his mom and dad. None of them wanted it, although nobody came out and said as much. So, they all just gritted their teeth and got on with it. Fourteen years to the month since leaving home to live on his own, Ryan found himself back in his cramped childhood bedroom, the same bed, the same sheets, the same desk, the same drapes, the same cupboard with the same rickety shelves. Nothing in the room had changed. Mom had been keeping it all for her grandchildren's sleepovers. Now he was reclaiming it instead. It felt wrong.

Ryan's parents were in their mid-50s and had blue-collar jobs. After they left for work each morning, a deep silence settled over their modest three-bedroom home. Ryan was alone with his thoughts, territory he would rather avoid. He felt trapped. During those first years back home, he aimlessly surfed the internet or sat by the window with a view to the street below and watched the world pass him by.

Such loneliness. Four walls hemmed him in. His mobile phone seldom rang. Occasionally, a friend would text him and they would go out for a beer. It seemed to him that those who still kept contact were the ones who were not embarrassed to be seen with him. He enjoyed the outing even if he dreaded getting there. But these excursions became fewer with time and then stopped. His social network, tied as it had been to a bar and drinking culture, had collapsed. As for women, there were none. Who was going to date a guy with no job, no money, who lived with his parents, struggled to walk, and occasionally wet himself? That is how he saw himself now.

Such loneliness. There were fragments of memories for company, the recollections of childhood triggered by being back in his old bedroom. Hours would drift by in reverie as he lay on his bed and relived great chunks of his life. School friends made and lost, his first cigarette, his first kiss, both disappointing, prank phone calls, stealing a pack of candies from the corner store, riding his bike, swimming in the public pool, the exams he never took seriously. Who could have predicted it would end up like this, being held prisoner by a body that would not obey his commands?

On his bedroom wall was a fading print of Renoir's *Luncheon of the Boating Party*. "How long has that been there?" he wondered aloud. "It was there before you were born," his mother snapped, "so much for your powers of observation." The news surprised him. He could not recall it. But now, with Ryan marooned, Renoir's masterpiece became the focus of his starved attention. Every aspect of the painting seemed to be the antithesis of his current existence: a happy social gathering outdoors on a boat, some water in the background, men and women, friends all, comfortable in their own company, a good lunch under the belt, and wine with it too, now onto fruit and desserts and the relaxed conversation that follows a good meal. The ages of the subjects were similar to his, he noted. And everyone in robust health! A golden moment in time, suffused with a contentment that was foreign to him now. Once upon a time he, too, had been able to meet with friends and drink and eat and laugh and flirt, and even if the location had been a little less classy than Renoir's boating scene, the emotions generated had been the same, the enjoyment surely no less keen. Now, as he saw it, MS had stripped him forever of such moments, confined them to a wistful longing and a vicarious pleasure kindled by the brushstrokes of an impressionist master. He should have hated that painting, he reasoned, for there, in those fading colors was so much in life that now seemed out of reach. If viewed this way, the painting was like a constant finger in the eye, a continual reminder of loss. Which is how he first saw the scene after belatedly becoming aware of it.

But then a strange thing happened. Once his mother had refused to remove the print, and harsh words were exchanged over this, Ryan's annoyance gradually gave way to acceptance and then pleasure. This transformation over the course of a year surprised him. He had even attached imaginary names to some of the subjects. Anglo-Canadian names, he laughed, like Todd, Scott, Connor, Erin, Kathy, and Krista. He would lose himself in daydreams about the luncheon party, insert himself into it, on occasion taking a chair alongside the woman with the glass of wine to her lips, the one not engaged in conversation, who perhaps was a little bored with the proceedings because none of the men present had captured her fancy.

Fantasy, daydreaming, an imaginary girlfriend—all were a refuge from the numbing loneliness that now defined his days. When he grew tired of the boating party and their perpetual bonhomie, frozen in time, he transferred his attentions online to Olga, an impossibly lithe and accommodating 24-year-old blonde graduate from the University of Belgorod in Russia, who notwithstanding her abundant charms, found herself inexplicably unattached and seeking a serious relationship with a man in the West. Olga was offering friendship and, as a bonus, should the relationship develop, a repertoire of carnal delights right out of Mata Hari's playbook. To a lonely young man stuck in his room, it seemed too good to be true, and it was of course. Ryan's mother, whose temperament was a mix of Calvinist morality, parsimony, and natural snoop, got wind of her son's internet infatuation with the gorgeous Olga, and while her son was in the bathroom one evening, slipped into his room and dealt it a death blow by informing the Belgorod bombshell that whatever meager financial resources her son had was from a government disability allowance, two-thirds of which automatically flowed into the family coffers to cover his living expenses, which by the way included budgeting for his adult diapers. Olga was neither seen nor heard from again. Ryan's fury was short-lived, although his humiliation lingered. But, at the end of the day, he had too many of his mother's genes not to know, deep down, that the internet relationship was nothing more than a scam. It had sure been fun, however, to play along for a while, if for no other reasons than Olga was infinitely pleasing on the eye and a lot more responsive than his fantasy girlfriend in the luncheon party.

Such loneliness. Once Renoir's boat slipped the moorings of his fraying attention and the family excitement over Olga subsided, Ryan's world seemed smaller than ever. He wondered, What now? Is this it? Is this as good as it gets? Hoping for no further physical deterioration, feeling grateful to some guiding hand—the neurologist's or a divine presence or both—that the wheelchair was not yet needed, nor the catheter or feeding tube? Winter found him completely housebound because of snow and ice. Summer was no better because of the heat. Spring and fall presented brief windows of opportunity to get out and about, but what was there to do? His friendships had dried up, his driver's license was suspended, and yes, there was public transport still available, albeit difficulty to use, but to what end? He had never been one to visit galleries and museums, or belong to a library. As for watching daytime television, well, he could not shake the conviction instilled by his family's strong work ethic that such an activity was slovenly. Ryan was thus a prisoner not only of his failing neurological function but also of his limited interests and rigid mindset. Trapped by these twin pincers, he could feel the walls calls close in still further.

It was at this point in his life, at his neurologist's firm recommendation, that Ryan came to see me. With access to his electronic medical records, I could follow the progression of his disease not only in the clinical case notes but also in his serial MRIs. There it was, in plain sight, the damage to his nervous system disseminated in time and place (figure 11.1). And with each progressive step toward further disability came the futile counterpunch of avoidant behavior. Commanding the moment was not an option at first, acceptance a long way off, but Ryan stuck at his psychotherapy, never missed an appointment, and gradually became increasingly comfortable with self-reflection. He came to see that in his loneliness, the young men and women of Renoir's boating party had become his surrogate companions, that he had been vulnerable to Olga's manipulations, and that he could not keep running from the reality of his situation. With that breakthrough, he was able to move on to the next phase in his therapy—planning, problem solving, and strategizing a way out of the cul-de-sac he had unwittingly entered.

In an incurable disease like multiple sclerosis, good symptom management from an interdisciplinary team and psychosocial support offer a solution to distressing shifts in time and space. Ryan's depression lifted with cognitive behavior therapy. His fatigue responded to long-acting

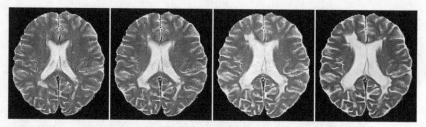

Figure 11.1. Serial MRI images showing a progressive increase in lesion burden and brain atrophy over 7.5 years. Images courtesy of Professor Arnold, McGill University and the Montreal Neurological Institute.

methylphenidate, a stimulant medication. His executive functioning remained relatively intact, even as his processing speed and working memory had slipped a little. With the assistance of his social worker, he obtained a transport pass for disabled people, a service funded by the government, which allowed him to attend a rehabilitation center, where he began exercising under supervision from a kinesiologist. He also started to attend a community center set up for people with disabilities. Here, he could swim, meet a peer group, relax with a cup of coffee, and chat with people just like himself without feeling self-conscious about his limitations. Before long, he was dating again, a woman who also had MS and who, like Ryan, had found herself isolated at home before her treatment team showed her a way out. Ryan was now out of the house four days a week. Each morning he would slide on his bottom down the stairs, unfold his collapsible walker, wait on the doorstep for his ride, and then get his day started with a workout. Saturday night was date night, his parents only too happy to fund a ride with a car service set up for people with disabilities. His social media connections now were with his girlfriend, a down-to-earth, sensible, and sensitive woman. Gone were the internet fantasies that preyed on his loneliness. For the first time in years, he could see a future for himself that did not look bleak.

Ryan's world began expanding again. Time quickened. There were activities to look forward to. A life once diminished—but with hope never extinguished—was rebuilt, painfully at first but, with each small success, joyously too.

1. The Paradox of Time and Space

1. Roberts A. *Churchill: Walking with Destiny*. London: Allen Lane; 2018.

2. Schumacher GA, Beebe G, Kibler RF, et al. Problems of experimental trials of therapy in multiple sclerosis: Report by the panel on the evaluation of experimental trials of therapy in multiple sclerosis. *Ann N Y Acad Sci*. 1965;122(1):552–568. https://doi.org/10.1111/j.1749-6632.1965.tb20235.x

3. Poser CM, Paty DW, Scheinberg L, et al. New diagnostic criteria for multiple sclerosis: Guidelines for research protocols. *Ann Neurol*. 1983;13:227–231. https://doi.org/10.1002/ana.410130302

4. McDonald WI, Compston A, Edan G, et al. Recommended diagnostic criteria for multiple sclerosis: Guidelines from the International Panel on the Diagnosis of Multiple Sclerosis. *Ann Neurol*. 2001;50:121–127. https://doi.org/10.1002/ana.1032

5. Polman CH, Reingold SC, Edan G, et al. Diagnostic criteria for multiple sclerosis: 2005 Revisions to the "McDonald Criteria." *Ann Neurol*. 2005;58:840–846. https://doi.org/10.1002/ana.20703

6. Polman CH, Reingold SC, Banwell B, et al. Diagnostic criteria for multiple sclerosis: 2010 revisions to the McDonald criteria. *Ann Neurol*. 2011;69(2):292–302. https://doi.org/10.1002/ana.22366

7. Thompson AJ, Banwell BL, Barkhof F, et al. Position Paper: Diagnosis of multiple sclerosis: 2017 revisions of the McDonald criteria. *Lancet Neurol*. 2018;17(2):162–173. https://doi.org/10.1016/S1474-4422(17)30470-2

8. Schaeffer J, Cossetti C, Mallucci G, Pluchino S. Multiple sclerosis. In: Zigmond MJ, Rowland LP, Coyle JT, eds. *Neurobiology of Brain Disorders*. Academic Press; 2015:497–520. https://doi.org/10.1016/B978-0-12-398270-4.00030-6

9. Ziemssen T, Tintoré M, de Moor C, et al. Cognitive and physical impairment in an MS population: Results from MS PATHS. *American Academy of Neurology Annual Meeting* 2020;P10.1-002.

10. Tremlett H, Paty D, Devonshire V. Disability progression in multiple sclerosis is slower than previously reported. *Neurology*. 2006;66(2):172–7. https://doi.org/10.1212/01.wnl.0000194259.90286.fe

11. Turcotte LA, Marrie RA, Patten SB, Hirdes JP. Clinical profile of persons with multiple sclerosis across the continuum of care. *Can J Neurol Sci*. 2018;45(2):188–198. https://doi.org/10.1017/cjn.2017.274

12. Marrie RA, Elliott L, Marriott J, et al. Effect of comorbidity on mortality in multiple sclerosis. *Neurology*. 2015;85(3):240–247. https://doi.org/10.1212/WNL .0000000000001718

13. Berger J, Demirel S. *What Time Is It?* Kendal, UK: Notting Hill Editions; 2019.

2. Cognition in General and Processing Speed in Particular

1. Charcot JM. *Lectures on the Diseases of the Nervous System delivered at the Salpetriere*. London: New Sydenham Society; 1877, 194–195.

2. Rao SM, Leo GJ, Bernardin L, Unverzagt F. Cognitive dysfunction in multiple sclerosis. I. Frequency, patterns, and prediction. *Neurology*. 1991;41(5):685–691. https://doi.org/10.1212/wnl.41.5.685

3. McIntosh-Michaelis SA, Roberts MH, Wilkinson SM, et al. The prevalence of cognitive impairment in a community survey of multiple sclerosis. *Br J Clin Psychol*. 1991;30(4):333–348. https://doi.org/10.1111/j.2044-8260.1991.tb00954.x

4. Kurtzke JF. Neurologic impairment in multiple sclerosis and the disability status scale. *Acta Neurol Scand*. 1970;46(4–5):493–512. https://doi.org/10.1111/j .1600-0404.1970.tb05808.x

5. Romero K, Shammi P, Feinstein A. Neurologists' accuracy in predicting cognitive impairment in multiple sclerosis. *Mult Scler Relat Disord*. 2015;4(4):291–295. https://doi.org/10.1016/j.msard.2015.05.009

6. Ruano L, Portaccio E, Goretti B, et al. Age and disability drive cognitive impairment in multiple sclerosis across disease subtypes. *Mult Scler*. 2017;23(9): 1258–1267. https://doi.org/10.1177/1352458516674367

7. Amato MP, Hakiki B, Goretti B, et al. Association of MRI metrics and cognitive impairment in radiologically isolated syndromes. *Neurology*. 2012;78(5):309–314. https://doi.org/10.1212/WNL.0b013e31824528c9

8. Amato MP, Ponziani G, Pracucci G, Bracco L, Siracusa G, Amaducci L. Cognitive impairment in early-onset multiple sclerosis: Pattern, predictors, and impact on everyday life in a 4-year follow-up. *Arch Neurol*. 1995;52(2):168–172. https://doi.org/10.1001/archneur.1995.00540260072019

9. Amato MP, Ponziani G, Siracusa G, Sorbi S. Cognitive dysfunction in early-onset multiple sclerosis: A reappraisal after 10 years. *Arch Neurol*. 2001;58(10):1602–1606. https://doi.org/10.1001/archneur.58.10.1602

10. Pardini M, Uccelli A, Grafman J, Yaldizli Ö, Mancardi G, Roccatagliata L. Isolated cognitive relapses in multiple sclerosis. *J Neurol Neurosurg Psychiatry*. 2014;85(9):1035–1037. https://doi.org/10.1136/jnnp-2013-307275

11. Benedict RHB, Morrow S, Rodgers J, et al. Characterizing cognitive function during relapse in multiple sclerosis. *Mult Scler J*. 2014;20(13):1745–1752. https://doi .org/10.1177/1352458514533229

12. Chiaravalloti ND, DeLuca J. Cognitive impairment in multiple sclerosis. *Lancet Neurol*. 2008;7(12):1139–1151. https://doi.org/10.1016/S1474-4422(08)70259-X

13. De Meo E, Portaccio E, Giogio A, et al. Identifying the distinct cognitive phenotypes in multiple sclerosis. *JAMA Neuroloy* 2021;78(4):414–425. https://doi .org/10.1001/jamaneurol.2020.4920

14. Clemens L, Langdon D. How does cognition relate to employment in multiple sclerosis? A systematic review. *Mult Scler Relat Disord*. 2018;26:183–191. https://doi .org/10.1016/j.msard.2018.09.018

15. van Gorp DAM, van der Hiele K, Heerings MAP, et al. Cognitive functioning as a predictor of employment status in relapsing-remitting multiple sclerosis: A 2-year longitudinal study. *Neurol Sci.* 2019;40(12):2555–2564. https://doi.org/10 .1007/s10072-019-03999-w

16. Rao SM, Leo GJ, Ellington L, Nauertz T, Bernardin L, Unverzagt F. Cognitive dysfunction in multiple sclerosis. II. Impact on employment and social functioning. *Neurology.* 1991;41(5):685–691. https://doi.org/10.1212/WNL.41.5.692

17. Wechsler D. *Wechsler Test of Adult Reading.* The Psychological Corporation; 2001.

18. Smith A. *Symbol Digit Modalities Test.* Los Angeles: Western Psychological Services; 1982.

19. Van Schependom J, D'hooghe MB, Cleynhens K, et al. The Symbol Digit Modalities Test as sentinel test for cognitive impairment in multiple sclerosis. *Eur J Neurol.* 2014;21(9):1219-e72. https://doi.org/10.1111/ene.12463

20. Benedict RH, Deluca J, Phillips G, LaRocca N, Hudson LD, Rudick R. Validity of the Symbol Digit Modalities Test as a cognition performance outcome measure for multiple sclerosis. *Mult Scler.* 2017;23(5):721–733. https://doi.org/10 .1177/1352458517690821

21. Benedict RHB, Weinstock-Guttman B, Fishman I, Sharma J, Tjoa CW, Bakshi R. Prediction of neuropsychological impairment in multiple sclerosis. *Arch Neurol.* 2004;61:226–230. https://doi.org/10.1001/archneur.61.2.226

22. Houtchens MK, Benedict RHB, Killiany R, et al. Thalamic atrophy and cognition in multiple sclerosis. *Neurology.* 2007;69:1213–1223. https://doi.org/10 .1212/01.wnl.0000276992.17011.b5

23. Benedict RHB, Bruce JM, Dwyer MG, et al. Neocortical atrophy, third ventricular width, and cognitive dysfunction in multiple sclerosis. *Arch Neurol.* 2006;63:1301–1306. https://doi.org/10.1001/archneur.63.9.1301

24. Silva PHR, Spedo CT, Barreira AA, Leoni RF. Symbol Digit Modalities Test adaptation for magnetic resonance imaging environment: A systematic review and meta-analysis. *Mult Scler Relat Disord.* 2018;20:136–143. https://doi.org/10.1016/j .msard.2018.01.014

25. Genova HM, Hillary FG, Wylie G, Rypma B, Deluca J. Examination of processing speed deficits in multiple sclerosis using functional magnetic resonance imaging. *J Int Neuropsychol Soc.* 2009;15(3):383–393. https://doi.org/10.1017 /S1355617709090535

26. Strober L, DeLuca J, Benedict RHB, et al. Symbol Digit Modalities Test: A valid clinical trial endpoint for measuring cognition in multiple sclerosis. *Mult Scler J.* 2019;25(13):1781–1790. https://doi.org/10.1177/1352458518808204

27. Gronwall D, Wrightson P. Delayed recovery of intellectual function after minor head injury. *Lancet.* 1974;304(7881):605–609. https://doi.org/10.1016/S0140 -6736(74)91939-4

28. Litvan I, Grafman J, Vendrell P, Martinez JM. Slowed information processing in multiple sclerosis. *Arch Neurol.* 1988;45(3):281–285. https://doi.org/10.1001 /archneur.1988.00520270059021

29. López-Góngora M, Querol L, Escartín A. A one-year follow-up study of the Symbol Digit Modalities Test (SDMT) and the Paced Auditory Serial Addition Test (PASAT) in relapsing-remitting multiple sclerosis: An appraisal of comparative

longitudinal sensitivity. *BMC Neurol.* 2015;15(1):40. https://doi.org/10.1186/s12883 -015-0296-2

30. Kalb R, Beier M, Benedict RHB, et al. Recommendations for cognitive screening and management in multiple sclerosis care. *Mult Scler J.* 2018;24(13):1665–1680. https://doi.org/10.1177/1352458518803785

31. Sandry J, Zuppichini M, Rothberg J, Valdespino-Hayden Z, DeLuca J. Poor encoding and weak early consolidation underlie memory acquisition deficits in multiple sclerosis: Retroactive interference, processing speed, or working memory? *Arch Clin Neuropsychol.* 2019;34(2):162–182. https://doi.org/10.1093/arclin /acy029

32. Rao SM. A manual for the Brief Repeatable Battery of Neuropsychological Tests in multiple sclerosis. *New York Natl Mult Scler Soc.* 1990.

33. Benedict RHB, Fischer JS, Archibald CJ, et al. Minimal neuropsychological assessment of MS patients: A consensus approach. *Clin Neuropsychol.* 2002;16(3): 381–397. https://doi.org/10.1076/clin.16.3.381.13859

34. Langdon DW, Amato MP, Boringa J, et al. Recommendations for a brief international cognitive assessment for multiple sclerosis (BICAMS). *Mult Scler J.* 2012;18(6):891–898. https://doi.org/10.1177/1352458511431076

35. Arnett P, Smith MM, Barwick FH, Benedict RHB, Ahlstrom BP. Oralmotor slowing in multiple sclerosis: Relationship to neuropsychological tasks requiring an oral response. *J Int Neuropsychol Soc.* 2008;14(3):454–462. https://doi.org/10.1017 /S1355617708080508

36. Friedova L, Rusz J, Motyl J, et al. Slowed articulation rate is associated with information processing speed decline in multiple sclerosis: A pilot study. *J Clin Neurosci.* 2019;65:28–33. https://doi.org/10.1016/j.jocn.2019.04.018

37. Bruce JM, Bruce AS, Arnett PA. Mild visual acuity disturbances are associated with performance on tests of complex visual attention in MS. *J Int Neuropsychol Soc.* 2007;13(3):544–548. https://doi.org/10.1017/S1355617707070658

38. Jacobs DA, Galetta SL. Multiple sclerosis and the visual system. *Ophthalmol Clin North Am.* 2004;17(3):265–273. https://doi.org/10.1016/j.ohc.2004.05.011

39. Frohman EM, Frohman TC, Zee DS, McColl R, Galetta S. The neuro-ophthalmology of multiple sclerosis. *Lancet Neurol.* 2005;4(2):111–121. https://doi .org/10.1016/S1474-4422(05)00992-0

40. Amezcua L, Morrow MJ, Jirawuthiworavong GV. Multiple sclerosis: Review of eye movement disorders and update of disease-modifying therapies. *Curr Opin Ophthalmol.* 2015;26(6):534–539. https://doi.org/10.1097/ICU .0000000000000211

41. Serra A, Chisari CG, Matta M. Eye movement abnormalities in multiple sclerosis: Pathogenesis, modeling, and treatment. *Front Neurol.* 2018;Feb 5;9:31. https://doi.org/10.3389/fneur.2018.00031

42. Fielding J, Kilpatrick T, Millist L, White O. Control of visually guided saccades in multiple sclerosis: Disruption to higher-order processes. *Neuropsychologia.* 2009;47(7):1647–1653. https://doi.org/10.1016/j.neuropsychologia.2009 .01.040

43. Fielding J, Kilpatrick T, Millist L, White O. Antisaccade performance in patients with multiple sclerosis. *Cortex.* 2009;45(7):900–903. https://doi.org/10.1016/j.cortex .2009.02.016

44. Fielding J, Kilpatrick T, Millist L, White O. Multiple sclerosis: Cognition and saccadic eye movements. *J Neurol Sci.* 2009;277(1–2):32–36. https://doi.org/10.1016/j.jns.2008.10.001

45. Kolbe SC, Kilpatrick TJ, Mitchell PJ, White O, Egan GF, Fielding J. Inhibitory saccadic dysfunction is associated with cerebellar injury in multiple sclerosis. *Hum Brain Mapp.* 2014;35(5):2310–2319. https://doi.org/10.1002/hbm.22329

46. Baner N, Schwarz C, Shaw M, et al. Speeded saccadic eye movement predicts symbol digit modalities test performance in multiple sclerosis. *Neurology.* 2017;88 (16 Supplement).

47. Pavisian B, Patel VP, Feinstein A. Cognitive mediated eye movements during the SDMT reveal the challenges with processing speed faced by people with MS. *BMC Neurol.* 2019;19(1):340. https://doi.org/10.1186/s12883-019-1543-8

48. Gill S, Santo J, Blair M, Morrow SA. Depressive symptoms are associated with more negative functional outcomes than anxiety symptoms in persons with multiple sclerosis. *J Neuropsychiatry Clin Neurosci.* 2019;31(1):37–42. https://doi.org/10.1176/appi.neuropsych.18010011

49. Leavitt VM, Brandstadter R, Fabian M, et al. Dissociable cognitive patterns related to depression and anxiety in multiple sclerosis. *Mult Scler J.* June 2019:26(10): 1247–1255. https://doi.org/10.1177/1352458519860319

50. Whitehouse CE, Fisk JD, Bernstein CN, et al. Comorbid anxiety, depression, and cognition in MS and other immune-mediated disorders. *Neurology.* 2019;92(5): E406-E417. https://doi.org/10.1212/WNL.0000000000006854

51. Rao SM, Leo GJ, St. Aubin-Faubert P. On the nature of memory disturbance in multiple sclerosis. *J Clin Exp Neuropsychol.* 1989;11(5):699–712. https://doi.org/10.1080/01688638908400926

52. Grafman J, Rao S, Bernardin L, Leo GJ. Automatic memory processes in patients with multiple sclerosis. *Arch Neurol.* 1991;48(10):1072–1075. https://doi.org/10.1001/archneur.1991.00530220094025

53. Krupp LB, Sliwinski M, Masur DM, Friedberg F, Coyle PK. Cognitive functioning and depression in patients with chronic fatigue syndrome and multiple sclerosis. *Arch Neurol.* 1994;51(7):705–710. https://doi.org/10.1001/archneur.1994.00540190089021

54. Fann JR, Uomoto JM, Katon WJ. Cognitive improvement with treatment of depression following mild traumatic brain injury. *Psychosomatics.* 2001;42(1):48–54. https://doi.org/10.1176/appi.psy.42.1.48

55. Castellano S, Ventimiglia A, Salomone S, et al. Selective serotonin reuptake inhibitors and serotonin and noradrenaline reuptake inhibitors improve cognitive function in partial responders depressed patients: Results from a prospective observational cohort study. *CNS Neurol Disord - Drug Targets.* 2016;15(10):1290–1298. https://doi.org/10.2174/1871527315666161003170312

56. Castellano S, Torrent C, Petralia MC, et al. Clinical and neurocognitive predictors of functional outcome in depressed patients with partial response to treatment: One year follow-up study. *Neuropsychiatr Dis Treat.* 2020;16:589–595. https://doi.org/10.2147/NDT.S224754

57. Patel VP, Walker LAS, Feinstein A. Deconstructing the Symbol Digit Modalities Test in multiple sclerosis: The role of memory. *Mult Scler Relat Disord.* 2017;17: 184–189. https://doi.org/10.1016/j.msard.2017.08.006

3. More on Processing Speed and the Tyranny of Distraction

1. Sumowski JF, Wylie GR, Deluca J, Chiaravalloti N. Intellectual enrichment is linked to cerebral efficiency in multiple sclerosis: Functional magnetic resonance imaging evidence for cognitive reserve. *Brain.* 2010;133(2):362–374. https://doi.org /10.1093/brain/awp307

2. Sumowski JF, Wylie GR, Gonnella A, Chiaravalloti N, Deluca J. Premorbid cognitive leisure independently contributes to cognitive reserve in multiple sclerosis. *Neurology.* 2010;75(16):1428–1431. https://doi.org/10.1212/WNL .0b013e3181f881a6

3. Sumowski JF, Rocca MA, Leavitt VM, et al. Reading, writing, and reserve: Literacy activities are linked to hippocampal volume and memory in multiple sclerosis. *Mult Scler.* 2016;22(12):1621–1625. https://doi.org/10.1177/1352458516630822

4. Benedict RHB, Morrow SA, Weinstock Guttman B, Cookfair D, Schretlen DJ. Cognitive reserve moderates decline in information processing speed in multiple sclerosis patients. *J Int Neuropsychol Soc.* 2010;16(5):829–835. https://doi.org/10 .1017/S1355617710000688

5. Patel VP, Zambrana A, Walker LA, Herrmann N, Feinstein A. Distraction adds to the cognitive burden in multiple sclerosis. *Mult Scler J.* 2017;23(1):106–113. https://doi.org/10.1177/1352458516641208

6. Feinstein A. Wordsworth, Bellow, and understanding multiple sclerosis. *Lancet Neurol.* June 2019. https://doi.org/10.1016/S1474-4422(19)30222-4

7. Patel VP, Zambrana A, Walker LA, Herrmann N, Swartz RH, Feinstein A. Distractibility in multiple sclerosis: The role of depression. *Mult Scler J - Exp Transl Clin.* 2016;2:2055217316653315. https://doi.org/10.1177/2055217316653150

8. Sadovnick AD, Remick RA, Allen J, et al. Depression and multiple sclerosis. *Neurology.* 1996;46(3):628–632. https://doi.org/10.1212/WNL.46.3.628

9. Patel VP, Walker L, Feinstein A. Processing speed and distractibility in multiple sclerosis: The role of sleep. *Mult Scler Relat Disord.* 2017;11:40–42. http://doi.org/10 .1016/j.msard.2016.11.012

10. Van der Stigchel S. *How Attention Works.* Cambridge, USA: The MIT Press; 2019. https://doi.org/10.7551/mitpress/11743.001.0001

11. Feinstein A, Lapshin H, O'Connor P. Looking anew at cognitive dysfunction in multiple sclerosis: The gorilla in the room. *Neurology.* 2012;79(11):1124–1129. https://doi.org/10.1212/WNL.0b013e3182698da3

12. Simons DJ, Chabris CF. Gorillas in our midst: Sustained inattentional blindness for dynamic events. *Perception.* 1999;28(9):1059–1074. https://doi.org/10 .1068/p2952

13. Rao SM, Losinski G, Mourany L, et al. Processing speed test: Validation of a self-administered, iPad®-based tool for screening cognitive dysfunction in a clinic setting. *Mult Scler.* 2017;23(14):1929–1937. https://doi.org/10.1177/1352458516688955

14. Patel VP, Shen L, Rose J, Feinstein A. Taking the tester out of the SDMT: A proof of concept fully automated approach to assessing processing speed in people with MS. *Mult Scler J.* 2019;25(11):1506–1513. https://doi.org/10.1177/1352458518792772

15. van Dongen L, Westerik B, van der Hiele K, et al. Introducing Multiple Screener: An unsupervised digital screening tool for cognitive deficits in MS. *Mult Scler Relat Disord.* 2020;38:101479. https://doi.org/10.1016/j.msard.2019 .101479

16. Wojcik CM, Beier M, Costello K, et al. Computerized neuropsychological assessment devices in multiple sclerosis: A systematic review. *Mult Scler J.* 2019;25(14): 1848–1869. https://doi.org/10.1177/1352458519879094

17. Landmeyer NC, Bürkner PC, Wiendl H, et al. Disease-modifying treatments and cognition in relapsing-remitting multiple sclerosis: A meta-analysis. *Neurology.* 2020;94(22):e2373–e2383. https://doi.org/10.1212/WNL.0000000000009522

18. Benedict RHB, Tomic D, Cree B, et al. Siponimod and cognition in secondary progressive multiple sclerosis: EXPAND secondary analyses. *Neurology* 2021;96(3): e376–e386. https://doi.org/10.1212/WNL.0000000000011275

19. Chen MH, Goverover Y, Genova HM, DeLuca J. Cognitive efficacy of pharmacologic treatments in multiple sclerosis: A systematic review. *CNS Drugs.* 2020;34(6):599–628. https://doi.org/10.1007/s40263-020-00734-4

20. Chan D, Binks S, Nicholas JM, et al. Effect of high-dose simvastatin on cognitive, neuropsychiatric and health-related quality of life measures in secondary progressive multiple sclerosis: Secondary analysis from the MS-STAT randomized, placebo controlled trial. *Lancet Neurology* 2017;16(8):591–600. https://doi.org/10.1016/S1474-4422(17)30113-8

21. Pedullà L, Brichetto G, Tacchino A, et al. Adaptive vs. non-adaptive cognitive training by means of a personalized App: A randomized trial in people with multiple sclerosis. *J Neuroeng Rehabil.* 2016;13(1):88. https://doi.org/10.1186/s12984-016-0193-y

22. Chiaravalloti ND, Goverover Y, Costa SL, DeLuca J. A pilot study examining speed of processing training (SPT) to improve processing speed in persons with multiple sclerosis. *Front Neurol.* 2018;(9):687. https://doi.org/10.3389/fneur.2018.00685

23. Messinis L, Nasios G, Kosmidis MH, et al. Efficacy of a computer-assisted cognitive rehabilitation intervention in relapsing-remitting multiple sclerosis patients: A multicenter randomized controlled trial. *Behav Neurol.* 2017:5919841. https://doi.org/10.1155/2017/5919841

24. Naeeni Davarani M, Arian Darestani A, Hassani-Abharian P, Vaseghi S, Zarrindast MR, Nasehi M. RehaCom rehabilitation training improves a wide-range of cognitive functions in multiple sclerosis patients. *Appl Neuropsychol.* 2020;5:1–11. https://doi.org/10.1080/23279095.2020.1747070

25. Messinis L, Kosmidis MH, Nasios G, et al. Do secondary progressive multiple sclerosis patients benefit from computer-based cognitive neurorehabilitation? A randomized sham controlled trial. *Mult Scler Relat Disord.* 2020;39:101932. https://doi.org/10.1016/j.msard.2020.101932

26. Barker L, Healy BC, Chan E, Leclaire K, Glanz BI. A pilot study to assess at-home speed of processing training for individuals with multiple sclerosis. *Mult Scler Int.* 2019;3;2019:3584259. https://doi.org/10.1155/2019/3584259

27. Bove RM, Rush G, Zhao C, et al. A videogame-based digital therapeutic to improve processing speed in people with multiple sclerosis: A feasibility study. *Neurol Ther.* 2019;8(1):135–145. https://doi.org/10.1007/s40120-018-0121-0

28. De Giglio L, De Luca F, Prosperini L, et al. A low-cost cognitive rehabilitation with a commercial video game improves sustained attention and executive functions in multiple sclerosis: A pilot study. *Neurorehabil Neural Repair.* 2015;29(5):453–461. https://doi.org/10.1177/1545968314554623

29. Maggio MG, Russo M, Cuzzola MF, et al. Virtual reality in multiple sclerosis rehabilitation: A review on cognitive and motor outcomes. *J Clin Neurosci.* 2019;65: 106–111. https://doi.org/10.1016/j.jocn.2019.03.017

30. DeLuca J, Chiaravalloti ND, Sandroff BM. Treatment and management of cognitive dysfunction in patients with multiple sclerosis. *Nat Rev Neurol.* 2020;16(6): 319–332. https://doi.org/10.1038/s41582-020-0355-1

31. Rosti-Otajärvi EM, Hämäläinen PI. Neuropsychological rehabilitation for multiple sclerosis. *Cochrane Database Syst Rev.* 2011. https://doi.org/10.1002 /14651858.cd009131.pub2

32. Rosti-Otajärvi EM, Hämäläinen PI. Neuropsychological rehabilitation for multiple sclerosis. *Cochrane Database Syst Rev.* 2014. https://doi.org/10.1002 /14651858.CD009131.pub3

33. Lampit A, Heine J, Finke C, et al. Computerized cognitive training in multiple sclerosis: A systematic review and meta-analysis. *Neurorehabil Neural Repair.* 2019;33(9):695–706. https://doi.org/10.1177/1545968319860490

4. Learning and Memory

1. Chiaravalloti ND, DeLuca J. Cognitive impairment in multiple sclerosis. *Lancet Neurol.* 2008;7(12):1139–1151. https://doi.org/10.1016/S1474-4422(08)70259-X

2. Baddeley A. Working memory: Looking back and looking forward. *Nat Rev Neurosci.* 2003;4(10):829–839. https://doi.org/10.1038/nrn1201

3. Wechsler D. *WAIS-R Manual: Wechsler Adult Intelligence Scale–Revised.* Psychological Corporation; 1981.

4. Gronwall D, Wrightson P. Delayed recovery of intellectual function after minor head injury. *Lancet.* 1974;304(7881):605–609. https://doi.org/10.1016/S0140 -6736(74)91939-4

5. Kirchner WK. Age differences in short-term retention of rapidly changing information. *J Exp Psychol.* 1958;55(4):352–358. https://doi.org/10.1037/h0043688

6. Owen AM, McMillan KM, Laird AR, Bullmore E. N-back working memory paradigm: A meta-analysis of normative functional neuroimaging studies. *Human Brain Mapping.* 2005;25:46–59. https://doi.org/10.1002/hbm.20131

7. Delis DC, Kramer JH, Kaplan E, Ober BA. *California Verbal Learning Test: Adult Version.* San Antonio, TX: The Psychological Corporation; 1987.

8. Buschke H, Fuld PA. Evaluating storage, retention, and retrieval in disordered memory and learning. *Neurology.* 1974;24(11):1019–1025. https://doi.org/10.1212 /wnl.24.11.1019

9. Benedict RHB, Munschauer F, Linn R, et al. Screening for multiple sclerosis cognitive impairment using a self-administered 15-item questionnaire. *Mult Scler.* 2003;9(1):95–101. https://doi.org/10.1191/1352458503ms861oa

10. Rao SM. Neuropsychology of multiple sclerosis: A critical review. *J Clin Exp Neuropsychol.* 1986;8(5):503–542. https://doi.org/10.1080/01688638608405173

11. Rao SM, Leo GJ, St. Aubin-Faubert P. On the nature of memory disturbance in multiple sclerosis. *J Clin Exp Neuropsychol.* 1989;11(5):699–712. https://doi.org /10.1080/01688638908400926

12. DeLuca J, Barbieri-Berger S, Johnson SK. The nature of memory impairments in multiple sclerosis: Acquisition versus retrieval. *J Clin Exp Neuropsychol.* 1994;16(2):183–189. https://doi.org/10.1080/01688639408402629

13. Sandry J, Zuppichini M, Rothberg J, Valdespino-Hayden Z, DeLuca J. Poor encoding and weak early consolidation underlie memory acquisition deficits in multiple sclerosis: Retroactive interference, processing speed, or working memory? *Arch Clin Neuropsychol.* 2019;34(2):162–182. https://doi.org/10.1093/arclin/acy029

14. Chiaravalloti ND, Moore NB, Nikelshpur OM, DeLuca J. An RCT to treat learning impairment in multiple sclerosis: The MEMREHAB trial. *Neurology.* 2013;81(24):2066–2072. https://doi.org/10.1212/01.wnl.0000437295.97946.a8

15. Thornton AE, Raz N, Tucker KA. Memory in multiple sclerosis: Contextual encoding deficits. *J Int Neuropsychol Soc.* 2002;8(3):395–409. https://doi.org/10.1017/S1355617702813200

16. Lafosse JM, Mitchell SM, Corboy JR, Filley CM. The nature of verbal memory impairment in multiple sclerosis: A list-learning and meta-analytic study. *J Int Neuropsychol Soc.* 2013;19(9):995–1008. https://doi.org/10.1017/S1355617713000957

17. Fink F, Eling P, Rischkau E, et al. The association between California Verbal Learning Test performance and fibre impairment in multiple sclerosis: Evidence from diffusion tensor imaging. *Mult Scler.* 2010;16(3):332–341. https://doi.org/10.1177/1352458509356367

18. Kutzelnigg A, Lassmann H. Cortical lesions and brain atrophy in MS. *J Neurol Sci.* 2005;233(1–2):55–59. https://doi.org/10.1016/j.jns.2005.03.027

19. Vercellino M, Masera S, Lorenzatti M, et al. Demyelination, inflammation, and neurodegeneration in multiple sclerosis deep gray matter. *J Neuropathol Exp Neurol.* 2009;68(5):489–502. https://doi.org/10.1097/NEN.0b013e3181a19a5a

20. Ramasamy DP, Benedict RHB, Cox JL, et al. Extent of cerebellum, subcortical and cortical atrophy in patients with MS. A case-control study. *J Neurol Sci.* 2009;282(1–2):47–54. https://doi.org/10.1016/j.jns.2008.12.034

21. Rocca MA, Mesaros S, Pagani E, Sormani MP, Comi G, Filippi M. Thalamic damage and long-term progression of disability in multiple sclerosis. *Radiology.* 2010;257(2):463–469. https://doi.org/10.1148/radiol.10100326

22. Minagar A, Barnett M, Benedict R, et al. The thalamus and multiple sclerosis. *Neurology.* 2013;80:210–219. https://doi.org/10.1212/WNL.0b013e31827b910b

23. Hulst HE, Geurts JJG. Gray matter imaging in multiple sclerosis: What have we learned? *BMC Neurol.* 2011;11:153. https://doi.org/10.1186/1471-2377-11-153

24. Gilmore CP, Donaldson I, Bö L, Owens T, Lowe J, Evangelou N. Regional variations in the extent and pattern of grey matter demyelination in multiple sclerosis: A comparison between the cerebral cortex, cerebellar cortex, deep grey matter nuclei and the spinal cord. *J Neurol Neurosurg Psychiatry.* 2009;80(2):182–187. https://doi.org/10.1136/jnnp.2008.148767

25. Calabrese M, Rinaldi F, Mattisi I, et al. The predictive value of gray matter atrophy in clinically isolated syndromes. *Neurology.* 2011;77(3):257–263. https://doi.org/10.1212/WNL.0b013e318220abd4

26. Rao SM, Glatt S, Hammeke TA, et al. Chronic progressive multiple sclerosis: Relationship between cerebral ventricular size and neuropsychological impairment. *Arch Neurol.* 1985;42(7):678–682. https://doi.org/10.1001/archneur.1985.04060070068018

27. Benedict RHB, Weinstock-Guttman B, Fishman I, Sharma J, Tjoa CW, Bakshi R. Prediction of neuropsychological impairment in multiple sclerosis. *Arch Neurol.* 2004;61:226–230. https://doi.org/10.1001/archneur.61.2.226

28. Houtchens MK, Benedict RHB, Killiany R, et al. Thalamic atrophy and cognition in multiple sclerosis. *Neurology.* 2007;69:1213–1223. https://doi.org/10.1212/01.wnl.0000276992.17011.b5

29. Zheng F, Cui D, Zhang L, et al. The volume of hippocampal subfields in relation to decline of memory recall across the adult lifespan. *Front Aging Neurosci.* 2018;10(OCT):320. https://doi.org/10.3389/fnagi.2018.00320

30. Geurts JJG, Bö L, Roosendaal SD, et al. Extensive hippocampal demyelination in multiple sclerosis. *J Neuropathol Exp Neurol.* 2007;66(9):819–827. https://doi.org/10.1097/nen.0b013e3181461f54

31. Papadopoulos D, Dukes S, Patel R, Nicholas R, Vora A, Reynolds R. Substantial archaeocortical atrophy and neuronal loss in multiple sclerosis. *Brain Pathol.* 2009;19(2):238–253. https://doi.org/10.1111/j.1750-3639.2008.00177.x

32. Dutta R, Chang A, Doud MK, et al. Demyelination causes synaptic alterations in hippocampi from multiple sclerosis patients. *Ann Neurol.* 2011;69(3):445–454. https://doi.org/10.1002/ana.22337

33. Koenig KA, Sakaie KE, Lowe MJ, et al. Hippocampal volume is related to cognitive decline and fornicial diffusion measures in multiple sclerosis. *Magn Reson Imaging.* 2014;32(4):354–358. https://doi.org/10.1016/j.mri.2013.12.012

34. Sicotte NL, Kern KC, Giesser BS, et al. Regional hippocampal atrophy in multiple sclerosis. *Brain.* 2008;131(4):1134–1141. https://doi.org/10.1093/brain/awn030

35. Planche V, Koubiyr I, Romero JE, et al. Regional hippocampal vulnerability in early multiple sclerosis: Dynamic pathological spreading from dentate gyrus to CA1. *Hum Brain Mapp.* 2018;39(4):1814–1824. https://doi.org/10.1002/hbm.23970

36. Longoni G, Rocca MA, Pagani E, et al. Deficits in memory and visuospatial learning correlate with regional hippocampal atrophy in MS. *Brain Struct Funct.* 2015;220(1):435–444. https://doi.org/10.1007/s00429-013-0665-9

37. Gold SM, Kern KC, O'Connor MF, et al. Smaller cornu ammonis 23/dentate gyrus volumes and elevated cortisol in multiple sclerosis patients with depressive symptoms. *Biol Psychiatry.* 2010;68(6):553–559. https://doi.org/10.1016/j.biopsych.2010.04.025

38. Koenig KA, Rao SM, Lowe MJ, et al. The role of the thalamus and hippocampus in episodic memory performance in patients with multiple sclerosis. *Mult Scler J.* 2019;25(4):574–584. https://doi.org/10.1177/1352458518760716

39. Llufriu S, Rocca MA, Pagani E, et al. Hippocampal-related memory network in multiple sclerosis: A structural connectivity analysis. *Mult Scler J.* 2019;25(6):801–810. https://doi.org/10.1177/1352458518771838

40. van Geest Q, Hulst HE, Meijer KA, Hoyng L, Geurts JJG, Douw L. The importance of hippocampal dynamic connectivity in explaining memory function in multiple sclerosis. *Brain Behav.* 2018;8(5):e00954. https://doi.org/10.1002/brb3.954

41. Chen MH, Goverover Y, Genova HM, DeLuca J. Cognitive efficacy of pharmacologic treatments in multiple sclerosis: A systematic review. *CNS Drugs.* 2020;34(6):599–628. https://doi.org/10.1007/s40263-020-00734-4

42. Aguirre N, Cruz-Gómez ÁJ, Miró-Padilla A, et al. Repeated working memory training improves task performance and neural efficiency in multiple sclerosis patients and healthy controls. *Mult Scler Int.* 2019;2019:2657902. https://doi.org/10.1155/2019/2657902

43. Covey TJ, Shucard JL, Benedict RH, Weinstock-Guttman B, Shucard DW. Improved cognitive performance and event-related potential changes following working memory training in patients with multiple sclerosis. *Mult Scler J - Exp Transl Clin.* 2018;4(1):2055217317747 62. https://doi.org/10.1177/2055217317747626

44. Chiaravalloti ND, Moore NB, DeLuca J. The efficacy of the modified Story Memory Technique in progressive MS. *Mult Scler J.* 2020;26(3):354–362. https://doi .org/10.1177/1352458519826463

45. Boukrina O, Dobryakova E, Schneider V, DeLuca J, Chiaravalloti ND. Brain activation patterns associated with paragraph learning in persons with multiple sclerosis: The MEMREHAB trial. *Int J Psychophysiol.* 2020;154:37–45. https://doi .org/10.1016/j.ijpsycho.2019.09.008

46. Chiaravalloti ND, Moore NB, Weber E, DeLuca J. The application of Strategy-based Training to Enhance Memory (STEM) in multiple sclerosis: A pilot RCT. *Neuropsychol Rehabil.* 2019:1–26. https://doi.org/10.1080/09602011.2019.1685550

47. Lincoln NB, Bradshaw LE, Constantinescu CS, et al. Cognitive rehabilitation for attention and memory in people with multiple sclerosis: A randomized controlled trial (CRAMMS). *Clin Rehabil.* 2020;34(2):229–241. https://doi.org/10.1177 /0269215519890378

48. das Nair R, Martin KJ, Lincoln NB. Memory rehabilitation for people with multiple sclerosis. *Cochrane Database Syst Rev.* 2016;(3). https://doi.org/10.1002 /14651858.CD008754.pub3

49. Darestani AA, Davarani MN, Hassani-Abharian P, Zarrindast M-R, Nas-ehi M. The therapeutic effect of treatment with RehaCom software on verbal performance in patients with multiple sclerosis. *J Clin Neurosci.* 2020;72:93–97. https://doi.org/10.1016/j.jocn.2020.01.007

50. Messinis L, Kosmidis MH, Nasios G, et al. Do secondary progressive multiple sclerosis patients benefit from computer-based cognitive neurorehabilitation? A randomized sham controlled trial. *Mult Scler Relat Disord.* 2020;39:101932. https://doi.org/10.1016/j.msard.2020.101932

51. Lampit A, Heine J, Finke C, et al. Computerized cognitive training in multiple sclerosis: A systematic review and meta-analysis. *Neurorehabil Neural Repair.* 2019;33(9):695–706. https://doi.org/10.1177/1545968319860490

52. Goodwin RA, Lincoln NB, das Nair R, Bateman A. Evaluation of NeuroPage as a memory aid for people with multiple sclerosis: A randomised controlled trial. *Neuropsychol Rehabil.* 2020;30(1):15–31. https://doi.org/10.1080/09602011.2018 .1447973

5. Planning and Problem Solving

1. Eling P, Derckx K, Maes R. On the historical and conceptual background of the Wisconsin Card Sorting Test. *Brain Cogn.* 2008. https://doi.org/10.1016/j.bandc .2008.01.006

2. Milner B. Effects of different brain lesions on card sorting: The role of the frontal lobes. *Arch Neurol.* 1963;9(1):90–100. https://doi.org/10.1001/archneur .1963.00460070100010

3. Heaton RK, Nelson LM, Thompson DS, Burks JS, Franklin GM. Neuropsychological findings in relapsing-remitting and chronic-progressive multiple sclerosis. *J Consult Clin Psychol.* 1985;53(1):103–110. https://doi.org/10.1037/0022-006X.53 .1.103

4. Beatty WW, Goodkin DE, Beatty PA, Monson N. Frontal lobe dysfunction and memory impairment in patients with chronic progressive multiple sclerosis. *Brain Cogn.* 1989;11(1):73–86. https://doi.org/10.1016/0278-2626(89)90006-7

5. Rao SM, Leo GJ, Bernardin L, Unverzagt F. Cognitive dysfunction in multiple sclerosis. I. Frequency, patterns, and prediction. *Neurology.* 1991;41(5):685–691. https://doi.org/10.1212/wnl.41.5.685

6. Delis DC, Squire LR, Bihrle A, Massman P. Componential analysis of problem-solving ability: Performance of patients with frontal lobe damage and amnesic patients on a new sorting test. *Neuropsychologia* 1992;30:683–697.

7. Delis, DC., Kaplan, E., Kramer J. *Examiner's Manual for the Delis-Kaplan Executive Function System.* 2001. https://doi.org/10.1080/09297040490911140

8. Benedict RHB. Integrating cognitive function screening and assessment into the routine care of multiple sclerosis patients. *CNS Spectr.* 2005;10(5):384–391. https://doi.org/10.1017/S1092852900022756

9. Stroop JR. Studies of interference in serial verbal reactions. *J Exp Psychol.* 1935;18(6):643–662. https://doi.org/10.1037/h0054651

10. Macniven JAB, Davis C, Ho MY, Bradshaw CM, Szabadi E, Constantinescu CS. Stroop performance in multiple sclerosis: Information processing, selective attention, or executive functioning? *J Int Neuropsychol Soc.* 2008;14(5):805–814. https://doi.org/10.1017/S1355617708080946

11. Denney DR, Lynch SG. The impact of multiple sclerosis on patients' performance on the Stroop Test: Processing speed versus interference. *J Int Neuropsychol Soc.* 2009;15(3):451–458. https://doi.org/10.1017/S1355617709090730

12. Lapshin H, Lanctôt KL, O'Connor P, Feinstein A. Assessing the validity of a computer-generated cognitive screening instrument for patients with multiple sclerosis. *Mult Scler J.* 2013;19(14):1905–1912. https://doi.org/10.1177/1352458513488841

13. Amato MP, Prestipino E, Bellinvia A, et al. Cognitive impairment in multiple sclerosis: An exploratory analysis of environmental and lifestyle risk factors. *PLoS One.* 2019;14(10). https://doi.org/10.1371/journal.pone.0222929

14. Goverover Y, Toglia J, DeLuca J. The weekly calendar planning activity in multiple sclerosis: A top-down assessment of executive functions. *Neuropsychol Rehabil.* 2020;30(7):1372–1387. https://doi.org/10.1080/09602011.2019.1584573

15. Leavitt VM, Wylie G, Krch D, Chiaravalloti N, DeLuca J, Sumowski JF. Does slowed processing speed account for executive deficits in multiple sclerosis? Evidence from neuropsychological performance and structural neuroimaging. *Rehabil Psychol.* 2014;59(4):422–8. https://doi.org/10.1037/a0037517

16. Genova HM, Deluca J, Chiaravalloti N, Wylie G. The relationship between executive functioning, processing speed, and white matter integrity in multiple sclerosis. *J Clin Exp Neuropsychol.* 2013;35(6):631–641. https://doi.org/10.1080/13803395.2013.806649

17. Roman CAF, Arnett PA. Structural brain indices and executive functioning in multiple sclerosis: A review. *J Clin Exp Neuropsychol.* 2016;38(3):261–274. https://doi.org/10.1080/13803395.2015.1105199

18. Dagenais E, Rouleau I, Tremblay A, et al. Role of executive functions in prospective memory in multiple sclerosis: Impact of the strength of cue-action association. *J Clin Exp Neuropsychol.* 2016;38(1):127–140. https://doi.org/10.1080/13803395.2015.1091063

19. Grech LB, Kiropoulos LA, Kirby KM, Butler E, Paine M, Hester R. Coping mediates and moderates the relationship between executive functions and psychological adjustment in multiple sclerosis. *Neuropsychology.* 2016;30(3):361–376. https://doi.org/10.1037/neu0000256

20. Grech LB, Kiropoulos LA, Kirby KM, Butler E, Paine M, Hester R. The effect of executive function on stress, depression, anxiety, and quality of life in multiple sclerosis. *J Clin Exp Neuropsychol.* 2015;37(5):549–562. https://doi.org/10.1080 /13803395.2015.1037723

21. Arnett PA, Higginson CI, Voss WD, et al. Depressed mood in multiple sclerosis: Relationship to capacity-demanding memory and attentional functioning. *Neuropsychology.* 1999;a13(3):434–446. https://doi.org/10.1037/0894-4105.13.3.434

22. Arnett PA, Higginson CI, Voss WD, Bender WI, Wurst JM, Tippin JM. Depression in multiple sclerosis: Relationship to working memory capacity. *Neuropsychology.* 1999;b13(4):546–556. https://doi.org/10.1037/0894-4105 .13.4.546

23. Demaree HA, Gaudino E, DeLuca J. The relationship between depressive symptoms and cognitive dysfunction in multiple sclerosis. *Cogn Neuropsychiatry.* 2003;8(3):161–171. https://doi.org/10.1080/13546800244000265

24. Parmenter BA, Zivadinov R, Kerenyi L, et al. Validity of the Wisconsin Card Sorting and Delis–Kaplan Executive Function System (DKEFS) sorting tests in multiple sclerosis. *J Clin Exp Neuropsychol.* 2007;29(2):215–223. https://doi.org/10 .1080/13803390600672163

25. Arnett PA, Rao SM, Bernardin L, Grafman J, Yetkin FZ, Lobeck L. Relationship between frontal lobe lesions and Wisconsin Card Sorting Test performance in patients with multiple sclerosis. *Neurology.* 1994;44(3):420–425. https://doi.org/10 .1212/wnl.44.3_part_1.420

26. Foong J, Rozewicz L, Quaghebeur G, et al. Executive function in multiple sclerosis. The role of frontal lobe pathology. *Brain.* 1997;120(1):15–26. https://doi .org/10.1093/brain/120.1.15

27. Cummings JL. Frontal-subcortical circuits and human behavior. *Arch Neurol.* 1993;50(8):873–880. https://doi.org/10.1001/archneur.1993.00540080076020

28. Geschwind N. Disconnexion syndromes in animals and man. *Brain.* 1965;88(2): 237–294. https://doi.org/10.1093/brain/88.2.237

29. Catani M, Ffytche DH. The rises and falls of disconnection syndromes. *Brain.* 2005;128(Pt 10):2224–2239. https://doi.org/10.1093/brain/awh622

30. Hubbard NA, Hutchison JL, Turner MP, et al. Asynchrony in executive networks predicts cognitive slowing in multiple sclerosis. *Neuropsychology.* 2016;30(1): 75–86. https://doi.org/10.1037/neu0000202

31. Koini M, Filippi M, Rocca MA, et al. Correlates of executive functions in multiple sclerosis based on structural and functional MR imaging: Insights from a multicenter study. *Radiology.* 2016;280(3):869–879. https://doi.org/10.1148/radiol .2016151809

32. Dobryakova E, Rocca MA, Valsasina P, et al. Abnormalities of the executive control network in multiple sclerosis phenotypes: An fMRI effective connectivity study. *Hum Brain Mapp.* 2016;37(6):2293–2304. https://doi.org/10.1002/hbm.23174

33. Gerstenecker A, Myers T, Lowry K, et al. Financial capacity and its cognitive predictors in progressive multiple sclerosis. *Arch Clin Neuropsychol.* 2017;32(8): 943–950. https://doi.org/10.1093/arclin/acx039

34. Tracy VL, Basso MR, Marson DC, Combs DR, Whiteside DM. Capacity for financial decision making in multiple sclerosis. *J Clin Exp Neuropsychol.* 2017;39(1): 46–57. https://doi.org/10.1080/13803395.2016.1201050

35. van Gorp DAM, van der Hiele K, Heerings MAP, et al. Cognitive functioning as a predictor of employment status in relapsing-remitting multiple sclerosis: A 2-year longitudinal study. *Neurol Sci.* 2019;40(12):2555–2564. https://doi.org/10 .1007/s10072-019-03999-w

36. Clemens L, Langdon D. How does cognition relate to employment in multiple sclerosis? A systematic review. *Mult Scler Relat Disord.* 2018;26:183–191. https://doi .org/10.1016/j.msard.2018.09.018

37. Chen MH, Goverover Y, Genova HM, DeLuca J. Cognitive efficacy of pharmacologic treatments in multiple sclerosis: A systematic review. *CNS Drugs.* 2020;34(6):599–628. https://doi.org/10.1007/s40263-020-00734-4

38. Fink F, Rischkau E, Butt M, Klein J, Eling P, Hildebrandt H. Efficacy of an executive function intervention programme in MS: A placebo-controlled and pseudo-randomized trial. *Mult Scler J.* 2010;16(9):1148–1151. https://doi.org/10 .1177/1352458510375440

39. Hanssen KT, Beiske AG, Landrø NI, Hofoss D, Hessen E. Cognitive rehabilitation in multiple sclerosis: A randomized controlled trial. *Acta Neurol Scand.* 2016;133(1):30–40. https://doi.org/10.1111/ane.12420

40. Messinis L, Nasios G, Kosmidis MH, et al. Efficacy of a computer-assisted cognitive rehabilitation intervention in relapsing-remitting multiple sclerosis patients: A multicenter randomized controlled trial. *Behav Neurol.* 2017. https://doi.org/10 .1155/2017/5919841

41. Angevaren M, Aufdemkampe G, Verhaar HJJ, Aleman A, Vanhees L. Physical activity and enhanced fitness to improve cognitive function in older people without known cognitive impairment. *Cochrane Database Syst Rev.* 2008;(2):CD005381. https://doi.org/10.1002/14651858.CD005381.pub2

42. Northey JM, Cherbuin N, Pumpa KL, Smee DJ, Rattray B. Exercise interventions for cognitive function in adults older than 50: A systematic review with meta-analysis. *Br J Sports Med.* 2018;52(3):154–160. https://doi.org/10.1136/bjsports -2016-096587

43. Song D, Yu DSF, Li PWC, Lei Y. The effectiveness of physical exercise on cognitive and psychological outcomes in individuals with mild cognitive impairment: A systematic review and meta-analysis. *Int J Nurs Stud.* 2018;79:155–164. https:// doi.org/10.1016/j.ijnurstu.2018.01.002

44. Loprinzi PD, Blough J, Ryu S, Kang M. Experimental effects of exercise on memory function among mild cognitive impairment: Systematic review and meta-analysis. *Phys Sportsmed.* 2019;47(1):21–26. https://doi.org/10.1080/00913847.2018 .1527647

45. Guure CB, Ibrahim NA, Adam MB, Said SM. Impact of physical activity on cognitive decline, dementia, and its subtypes: Meta-analysis of prospective studies. *Biomed Res Int.* 2017;2017. https://doi.org/10.1155/2017/9016924

46. Du Z, Li Y, Li J, Zhou C, Li F, Yang X. Physical activity can improve cognition in patients with Alzheimer's disease: A systematic review and meta-analysis of randomized controlled trials. *Clin Interv Aging.* 2018;13:1593–1603. https://doi.org /10.2147/CIA.S169565

47. Zheng G, Zhou W, Xia R, Tao J, Chen L. Aerobic exercises for cognition rehabilitation following stroke: A systematic review. *J Stroke Cerebrovasc Dis.* 2016;25(11):2780–2789. https://doi.org/10.1016/j.jstrokecerebrovasdis.2016.07.035

48. Vanderbeken I, Kerckhofs E. A systematic review of the effect of physical exercise on cognition in stroke and traumatic brain injury patients. *NeuroRehabilitation.* 2017;40(1):33–48. https://doi.org/10.3233/NRE-161388

49. Pajonk FG, Wobrock T, Gruber O, et al. Hippocampal plasticity in response to exercise in schizophrenia. *Arch Gen Psychiatry.* 2010;67(2):133–143. https://doi.org/10.1001/archgenpsychiatry.2009.193

50. Kjølhede T, Siemonsen S, Wenzel D, et al. Can resistance training impact MRI outcomes in relapsing-remitting multiple sclerosis? *Mult Scler J.* 2018;24(10): 1356–1365. https://doi.org/10.1177/1352458517722645

51. Orban A, Garg B, Sammi MK, et al. Effect of high-intensity exercise on multiple sclerosis function and phosphorous magnetic resonance spectroscopy outcomes. *Med Sci Sports Exerc.* 2019;51(7):1380–1386. https://doi.org/10.1249/MSS.0000000000001914

52. Gharakhanlou R, Wesselmann L, Rademacher A, et al. Exercise training and cognitive performance in persons with multiple sclerosis: A systematic review and multilevel meta-analysis of clinical trials. *Mult Scler.* May 2020. https://doi.org/10.1177/1352458520917935

53. Feinstein A, Freeman J, Lo AC. Treatment of progressive multiple sclerosis: What works, what does not, and what is needed. *Lancet Neurol.* 2015;14(2):194–207. https://doi.org/10.1016/S1474-4422(14)70231-5

54. Feinstein A, Amato MP, Brichetto G, et al. Study protocol: Improving cognition in people with progressive multiple sclerosis: A multi-arm, randomized, blinded, sham-controlled trial of cognitive rehabilitation and aerobic exercise (COGEx). *BMC Neurol.* 2020;20(1):204. https://doi.org/10.1186/s12883-020-01772-7

55. Jiménez-Morales RM, Herrera-Jiménez LF, Macías-Delgado Y, Pérez-Medinilla YT, Díaz-Díaz SM, Forn C. Cognitive training combined with aerobic exercises in multiple sclerosis patients: A pilot study. *Rev Neurol.* 2017;64(11):489–495. https://doi.org/10.33588/rn.6411.2016312

6. *Global Impairment and the Unraveling of Personality*

1. Ruano L, Portaccio E, Goretti B, et al. Age and disability drive cognitive impairment in multiple sclerosis across disease subtypes. *Mult Scler.* 2017;23(9): 1258–1267. https://doi.org/10.1177/1352458516674367

2. Krupp LB, Christodoulou C, Melville P, Scherl WF, MacAllister WS, Elkins LE. Donepezil improved memory in multiple sclerosis in a randomized clinical trial. *Neurology.* 2004;63(9):1579–1585. https://doi.org/10.1212/01.WNL.0000142989.09633.5A

3. Krupp LB, Christodoulou C, Melville P, et al. Multicenter randomized clinical trial of donepezil for memory impairment in multiple sclerosis. *Neurology.* 2011;76(11): 1500–1507. https://doi.org/10.1212/WNL.0b013e318218107a

4. Greene YM, Tariot PN, Wishart H, et al. A 12-week, open trial of donepezil hydrochloride in patients with multiple sclerosis and associated cognitive impairments. *J Clin Psychopharmacol.* 2000;20(3):350–356. https://doi.org/10.1097/00004714-200006000-00010

5. Mischel W. *Personality and Assessment*. New York: John Wiley & Sons; 1968.

6. Schwartz L, Kraft GH. The role of spouse responses to disability and family environment in multiple sclerosis. *Am J Phys Med Rehabil*. 1999;78(6):525–532. https://doi.org/10.1097/00002060-199911000-00006

7. Uccelli MM. The impact of multiple sclerosis on family members: A review of the literature. *Neurodegener Dis Manag*. 2014;4(2):177–185. https://doi.org/10.2217/nmt.14.6

8. Petrikis P, Baldouma A, Katsanos AH, Konitsiotis S, Giannopoulos S. Quality of life and emotional strain in caregivers of patients with multiple sclerosis. *J Clin Neurol*. 2019;15(1):77–83. https://doi.org/10.3988/jcn.2019.15.1.77

9. Pahlavanzadeh S, Dalvi-Isfahani F, Alimohammadi N, Chitsaz A. The effect of group psycho-education program on the burden of family caregivers with multiple sclerosis patients in Isfahan in 2013–2014. *Iran J Nurs Midwifery Res*. 2015;20(4): 420–425. https://doi.org/10.4103/1735-9066.161000

10. Marin RS, Biedrzycki RC, Firinciogullari S. Reliability and validity of the apathy evaluation scale. *Psychiatry Res*. 1991;38(2);143–162. https://doi.org/10.1016/0165-1781(91)90040-V

11. Marin RS. Differential diagnosis and classification of apathy. *Am J Psychiatry*. 1990;147(1):22–30. https://doi.org/10.1176/ajp.147.1.22

12. Marin RS. Apathy: A neuropsychiatric syndrome. *J Neuropsychiatry Clin Neurosci*. 1991;3(3):243–254. https://doi.org/10.1176/jnp.3.3.243

13. Cummings JL. Frontal-subcortical circuits and human behavior. *Arch Neurol*. 1993;50(8):873–880. https://doi.org/10.1001/archneur.1993.00540080076020

14. American Psychological Association (APA). Personality Disorders. In: *Diagnostic and Statistical Manual of Mental Disorders*. 5th ed. Washington, DC: American Psychiatric Association; 2013.

15. Costa PT, McCrae RR. *Professional Manual for the Revised NEO Personality Inventory and NEO Five-Factor Inventory*. Odessa, FL: Psychological Assessment Resources Inc.; 1992.

16. Roy S, Schwartz CE, Duberstein P, et al. Synergistic effects of reserve and adaptive personality in multiple sclerosis. *J Int Neuropsychol Soc*. 2016;22(9):920–927. https://doi.org/10.1017/S1355617716000333

17. Roy S, Drake AS, Eizaguirre MB, et al. Trait neuroticism, extraversion, and conscientiousness in multiple sclerosis: Link to cognitive impairment? *Mult Scler*. 2018;24(2):205–213. https://doi.org/10.1177/1352458517695467

18. Leavitt VM, Buyukturkoglu K, Inglese M, Sumowski JF. Protective personality traits: High openness and low neuroticism linked to better memory in multiple sclerosis. *Mult Scler*. 2017;23(13):1786–1790. https://doi.org/10.1177/1352458516685417

19. Benedict RHB, Schwartz CE, Duberstein P, et al. Influence of personality on the relationship between gray matter volume and neuropsychiatric symptoms in multiple sclerosis. *Psychosom Med*. 2013;75(3):253–261. https://doi.org/10.1097/PSY.0b013e31828837cc

20. Rabins PV, Brooks BR, O'Donnell P, et al. Structural brain correlates of emotional disorder in multiple sclerosis. *Brain*. 1986;109(4):585–597. https://doi.org/10.1093/brain/109.4.585

21. Roy S, Rodgers J, Drake AS, Zivadinov R, Weinstock-Guttman B, Benedict RHB. Stable neuropsychiatric status in multiple sclerosis: A 3-year study. *Mult Scler*. 2016;22(4):569–574. https://doi.org/10.1177/1352458515597570

22. Roy S, Drake A, Fuchs T, et al. Longitudinal personality change associated with cognitive decline in multiple sclerosis. *Mult Scler J.* 2018;24(14):1909–1912. https://doi.org/10.1177/1352458517753720

23. Tang TZ, DeRubeis RJ, Hollon SD, Amsterdam J, Shelton R, Schalet B. Personality change during depression treatment: A placebo-controlled trial. *Arch Gen Psychiatry.* 2009;66(12):1322–1330. https://doi.org/10.1001/archgenpsychiatry .2009.166

24. Krasner MS, Epstein RM, Beckman H, et al. Association of an educational program in mindful communication with burnout, empathy, and attitudes among primary care physicians. *JAMA - J Am Med Assoc.* 2009;302(12):1284–1293. https://doi.org/10.1001/jama.2009.1384

7. Sadness and Irritability

1. Minden SL, Orav J, Reich P. Depression in multiple sclerosis. *Gen Hosp Psychiatry.* 1987;9(6):426–434. https://doi.org/10.1016/0163-8343(87)90052-1

2. Joffe RT, Lippert GP, Gray TA, Sawa G, Horvath Z. Personal and family history of affective illness in patients with multiple sclerosis. *J Affect Disord.* 1987;12(1):63–65. https://doi.org/10.1016/0165-0327(87)90062-0

3. Sadovnick AD, Remick RA, Allen J, et al. Depression and multiple sclerosis. *Neurology.* 1996;46(3):628–632. https://doi.org/10.1212/WNL.46.3.628

4. Patten SB, Beck CA, Williams JVA, Barbui C, Metz LM. Major depression in multiple sclerosis: A population-based perspective. *Neurology.* 2003;61(11):1524–1527. https://doi.org/10.1212/01.WNL.0000095964.34294.B4

5. Marrie RA, Fisk JD, Tremlett H, Wolfson C, Warren S, Tennakoon A, Leung S, Patten S. Differences in the burden of psychiatric comorbidity in MS vs the general population. *Neurology.* 2015;85(22):1972–1979. https://doi.org/10.1212/WNL .0000000000002174

6. Marrie RA, Elliott L, Marriott J, et al. Effect of comorbidity on mortality in multiple sclerosis. *Neurology.* 2015;85(3):240–247. https://doi.org/10.1212/WNL .0000000000001718

7. McDonald WI. The significance of optic neuritis. *Trans Ophthalmol Soc UK.* 1983;103:230–246.

8. Mohr DC, Goodkin DE, Gatto N, Van Der Wende J. Depression, coping and level of neurological impairment in multiple sclerosis. *Mult Scler J.* 1997;3(4):254–258. https://doi.org/10.1177/135245859700300408

9. Rommer PS, Sühnel A, König N, Zettl UK. Coping with multiple sclerosis—the role of social support. *Acta Neurol Scand.* 2017;136(1):11–16. https://doi.org/10 .1111/ane.12673

10. Lorefice L, Fenu G, Frau J, Coghe G, Marrosu MG, Cocco E. The burden of multiple sclerosis and patients' coping strategies. *BMJ Support Palliat Care.* 2018;8(1): 38–40. https://doi.org/10.1136/bmjspcare-2017-001324

11. Arnett PA, Higginson CI, Voss WD, Randolph JJ, Grandey AA. Relation-ship between coping, cognitive dysfunction and depression in multiple sclerosis. *Clin Neuropsychol.* 2002;16(3):341–355. https://doi.org/10.1076/clin.16.3.341 .13852

12. Grytten N, Skår AB, Aarseth JH, et al. The influence of coping styles on long-term employment in multiple sclerosis: A prospective study. *Mult Scler.* 2017;23(7):1008–1017. https://doi.org/10.1177/1352458516667240

13. Strober LB, Chiaravalloti N, DeLuca J. Should I stay or should I go? A prospective investigation examining individual factors impacting employment status among individuals with multiple sclerosis (MS). *Work*. 2018;59(1):39–47. https://doi.org/10.3233/WOR-172667

14. Stolove CA, Galatzer-Levy IR, Bonanno GA. Emergence of depression following job loss prospectively predicts lower rates of reemployment. *Psychiatry Res*. 2017;253:79–83. https://doi.org/10.1016/j.psychres.2017.03.036

15. Zuelke AE, Luck T, Schroeter ML, et al. The association between unemployment and depression—results from the population-based LIFE-adult-study. *J Affect Disord*. 2018;235:399–406. https://doi.org/10.1016/j.jad.2018.04.073

16. Lode K, Bru E, Klevan G, Myhr KM, Nyland H, Larsen JP. Depressive symptoms and coping in newly diagnosed patients with multiple sclerosis. *Mult Scler*. 2009;15(5):638–643. https://doi.org/10.1177/1352458509102313

17. McCabe MP, McKern S, McDonald E. Coping and psychological adjustment among people with multiple sclerosis. *J Psychosom Res*. 2004;56(3):355–361. https://doi.org/10.1016/S0022-3999(03)00132-6

18. Arnett PA, Randolph JJ. Longitudinal course of depression symptoms in multiple sclerosis. *J Neurol Neurosurg Psychiatry*. 2006;77(5):606–610. https://doi.org/10.1136/jnnp.2004.047712

19. Tan-Kristanto S, Kiropoulos LA. Resilience, self-efficacy, coping styles and depressive and anxiety symptoms in those newly diagnosed with multiple sclerosis. *Psychol Heal Med*. 2015;20(6):635–645. https://doi.org/10.1080/13548506.2014.999810

20. Roubinov DS, Turner AP, Williams RM. Coping among individuals with multiple sclerosis: Evaluating a goodness-of-fit model. *Rehabil Psychol*. 2015;60(2):162–168. https://doi.org/10.1037/rep0000032

21. Moreau T, Bungener C, Heinzlef O, et al. Anxiety and coping strategy changes in multiple sclerosis patients initiating fingolimod: The GRACE prospective study. *Eur Neurol*. 2017;77(1–2):47–55. https://doi.org/10.1159/000451077

22. Keramat Kar M, Whitehead L, Smith CM. Characteristics and correlates of coping with multiple sclerosis: A systematic review. *Disabil Rehabil*. 2019;41(3):250–264. https://doi.org/10.1080/09638288.2017.1387295

23. Wilski M, Gabryelski J, Brola W, Tomasz T. Health-related quality of life in multiple sclerosis: Links to acceptance, coping strategies and disease severity. *Disabil Health J*. 2019;12(4):608–614. https://doi.org/10.1016/j.dhjo.2019.06.003

24. Bandura A. Self-efficacy: Toward a unifying theory of behavioral change. *Psychological Review* 1977;84(2):191–215.

25. Schwartz CE, Coulthard-Morris L, Zeng Q, Retzlaff P. Measuring self-efficacy in people with multiple sclerosis: A validation study. *Arch Phys Med Rehabil*. 1996;77(4):394–398. https://doi.org/10.1016/S0003-9993(96)90091-X

26. Airlie J, Baker GA, Smith SJ, Young CA. Measuring the impact of multiple sclerosis on psychosocial functioning: The development of a new self-efficacy scale. *Clin Rehabil*. 2001;15(3):259–265. https://doi.org/10.1191/026921501668362643

27. Rigby SA, Domenech C, Thornton EW, Tedman S, Young CA. Development and validation of a self-efficacy measure for people with multiple sclerosis: The multiple sclerosis self-efficacy scale. *Mult Scler*. 2003;9(1):73–81. https://doi.org/10.1191/1352458503ms870oa

28. Young CA, Mills RJ, Woolmore J, Hawkins CP, Tennant A. The unidimensional self-efficacy scale for MS (USE-MS): Developing a patient based and patient reported outcome. *Mult Scler J.* 2012;18(9):1326–1333. https://doi.org/10.1177 /1352458512436592

29. Stuifbergen AK, Becker H, Blozis S, Timmerman G, Kullberg V. A randomized clinical trial of a wellness intervention for women with multiple sclerosis. *Arch Phys Med Rehabil.* 2003;84(4):467–476. https://doi.org/10.1053/apmr.2003.50028

30. Motl RW, McAuley E, Snook EM, Gliottoni RC. Physical activity and quality of life in multiple sclerosis: Intermediary roles of disability, fatigue, mood, pain, self-efficacy and social support. *Psychol Heal Med.* 2009;14(1):111–124. https://doi .org/10.1080/13548500802241902

31. Schmitt MM, Goverover Y, DeLuca J, Chiaravalloti N. Self-efficacy as a predictor of self-reported physical, cognitive, and social functioning in multiple sclerosis. *Rehabil Psychol.* 2014;59(1):27–34. https://doi.org/10.1037/a0035288

32. Tamar Kalina J, Hinojosa J, Strober L, Bacon J, Donnelly S, Goverover Y. Randomized controlled trial to improve self-efficacy in people with multiple sclerosis: The community reintegration for socially isolated patients (CRISP) program. *Am J Occup Ther.* 2018;72(5):7205205030p1–7205205030p8. https://doi.org/10.5014 /ajot.2018.026864

33. Strober LB. Quality of life and psychological well-being in the early stages of multiple sclerosis (MS): Importance of adopting a biopsychosocial model. *Disabil Health J.* 2018;11(4):555–561. https://doi.org/10.1016/j.dhjo.2018.05.003

34. Koelmel E, Hughes AJ, Alschuler KN, Ehde DM. Resilience mediates the longitudinal relationships between social support and mental health outcomes in multiple sclerosis. *Arch Phys Med Rehabil.* 2017;98(6):1139–1148. https://doi.org /10.1016/j.apmr.2016.09.127

35. Gromisch ES, Sloan J, Zemon V, et al. Development of the Multiple Sclerosis Resiliency Scale (MSRS). *Rehabil Psychol.* 2018;63(3):357–364. https://doi.org/10 .1037/rep0000219

36. Koch MW, Glazenborg A, Uyttenboogaart M, Mostert J, De Keyser J. Pharmacologic treatment of depression in multiple sclerosis. *Cochrane Database Syst Rev.* 2011;(2). https://doi.org/10.1002/14651858.cd007295.pub2

37. Schiffer RB, Wineman NM. Antidepressant pharmacotherapy of depression associated with multiple sclerosis. *Am J Psychiatry.* 1990;147(11):1493–1497. https://doi.org/10.1176/ajp.147.11.1493

38. Ehde DM, Kraft GH, Chwastiak L, et al. Efficacy of paroxetine in treating major depressive disorder in persons with multiple sclerosis. *Gen Hosp Psychiatry.* 2008;30(1):40–48. https://doi.org/10.1016/j.genhosppsych.2007.08.002

39. Mohr DC, Boudewyn AC, Goodkin DE, Bostrom A, Epstein L. Comparative outcomes for individual cognitive-behavior therapy, supportive-expressive group psychotherapy, and sertraline for the treatment of depression in multiple sclerosis. *J Consult Clin Psychol.* 2001;69(6):942–949. https://doi.org/10.1037/0022-006X .69.6.942

40. Flax JW, Gray J, Herbert J. Effect of fluoxetine on patients with multiple sclerosis. *Am J Psychiatry.* 1991;148(11):1603. https://doi.org/10.1176/ajp.148.11.1603a

41. Bayas A, Schuh K, Baier M, et al. Combination treatment of fingolimod with antidepressants in relapsing-remitting multiple sclerosis patients with depression: A

multicentre, open-label study—REGAIN. *Ther Adv Neurol Disord.* 2016;9(5):378–388. https://doi.org/10.1177/1756285616651197

42. Scott TF, Nussbaum P, McConnell H, Brill P. Measurement of treatment response to sertraline in depressed multiple sclerosis patients using the Carroll scale. *Neurol Res.* 1995;17(6):421–422. https://doi.org/10.1080/01616412.1995.11740355

43. Barak Y, Ur E, Achiron A. Moclobemide treatment in multiple sclerosis patients with comorbid depression: An open-label safety trial. *J Neuropsychiatry Clin Neurosci.* 1999;11(2):271–273. https://doi.org/10.1176/jnp.11.2.271

44. Kessler TM, Fowler CJ, Panicker JN. Sexual dysfunction in multiple sclerosis. *Expert Rev Neurother.* 2009;9(3):341–350. https://doi.org/10.1586/14737175.9.3.341

45. Marck CH, Jelinek PL, Weiland TJ, et al. Sexual function in multiple sclerosis and associations with demographic, disease and lifestyle characteristics: An international cross-sectional study. *BMC Neurol.* 2016;16(1):210. https://doi.org/10.1186/s12883-016-0735-8

46. Nathoo N, Mackie A. Treating depression in multiple sclerosis with antidepressants: A brief review of clinical trials and exploration of clinical symptoms to guide treatment decisions. *Mult Scler Relat Disord.* 2017;18:177–180. https://doi.org/10.1016/j.msard.2017.10.004

47. Harrison JE, Lophaven S, Olsen CK. Which cognitive domains are improved by treatment with vortioxetine? *Int J Neuropsychopharmacol.* 2016;19(10):1–6. https://doi.org/10.1093/ijnp/pyw054

48. McIntyre R, Harrison J, Loft H, Jacobson W, Olsen C. The effects of vortioxetine on cognitive function in patients with major depressive disorder: A meta-analysis of three randomized controlled trials. *Int J Neuropsychopharmacol.* 2016;19(10): pyw055. https://doi.org/10.1093/ijnp/pyw055

49. Mohr DC, Likosky W, Bertagnolli A, Goodkin DE, Van Der Wende J, Dwyer P, Dick LP. Telephone-administered cognitive-behavioral therapy for the treatment of depressive symptoms in multiple sclerosis. *J. Consulting Clinical Psychology* 2000;68(2): 356–61. https://doi.org/10.1037/0022-006x.68.2.356

50. Mohr DC, Hart SL, Julian L, et al. Telephone-administered psychotherapy for depression. *Arch Gen Psychiatry.* 2005;62(9):1007–1014. https://doi.org/10.1001/archpsyc.62.9.1007

51. Kiropoulos LA, Kilpatrick T, Holmes A, Threader J. A pilot randomized controlled trial of a tailored cognitive behavioural therapy based intervention for depressive symptoms in those newly diagnosed with multiple sclerosis. *BMC Psychiatry.* 2016;16(1):435. https://doi.org/10.1186/s12888-016-1152-7

52. Kiropoulos L, Kilpatrick T, Kalincek T, et al. Comparison of the effectiveness of a tailored cognitive behavioural therapy with a supportive listening intervention for depression in those newly diagnosed with multiple sclerosis (the ACTION-MS trial): Protocol of an assessor-blinded, active comparator randomised control trial. *Trials* 2020;21(100). https://doi.org/10.1186/s13063-019-4018-8

53. Forman AC, Lincoln NB. Evaluation of an adjustment group for people with multiple sclerosis: A pilot randomized controlled trial. *Clin Rehabil.* 2010;24(3): 211–221. https://doi.org/10.1177/0269215509343492

54. Lincoln NB, Yuill F, Holmes J, et al. Evaluation of an adjustment group for people with multiple sclerosis and low mood: A randomized controlled trial. *Mult Scler J.* 2011;17(10):1250–1257. https://doi.org/10.1177/1352458511408753

55. Ratajska A, Zurawski J, Healy B, Glanz BI. Computerized cognitive behavioral therapy for treatment of depression in multiple sclerosis: A narrative review of current findings and future directions. *Int J MS Care*. 2019;21(3):113–123. https://doi.org/10.7224/1537-2073.2017-094

56. Siengsukon CF, Alshehri M, Williams C, Drerup M, Lynch S. Feasibility and treatment effect of cognitive behavioral therapy for insomnia in individuals with multiple sclerosis: A pilot randomized controlled trial. *Mult Scler Relat Disord*. 2020;40. https://doi.org/10.1016/j.msard.2020.101958

57. Ehde DM, Alschuler KN, Day MA, et al. Mindfulness-based cognitive therapy and cognitive behavioral therapy for chronic pain in multiple sclerosis: A randomized controlled trial protocol. *Trials*. 2019;20(1):774. https://doi.org/10.1186/s13063-019-3761-1

58. Gromisch ES, Kerns RD, Czlapinski R, et al. Cognitive behavioral therapy for the management of multiple sclerosis-related pain: A randomized clinical trial. *Int J MS Care*. 2020;22(1):8–14. https://doi.org/10.7224/1537-2073.2018-023

59. Chalah MA, Ayache SS. Cognitive behavioral therapies and multiple sclerosis fatigue: A review of literature. *J Clin Neurosci*. 2018;52:1–4. https://doi.org/10.1016/j.jocn.2018.03.024

60. Richards DA, Ekers D, McMillan D, et al. Cost and outcome of behavioural activation versus cognitive behavioural therapy for depression (COBRA): A randomised, controlled, non-inferiority trial. *Lancet*. 2016;388(10047):871–880. https://doi.org/10.1016/S0140-6736(16)31140-0

61. Turner AP, Hartoonian N, Hughes AJ, et al. Physical activity and depression in MS: The mediating role of behavioral activation. *Disabil Health J*. 2019;12(4):635–640. https://doi.org/10.1016/j.dhjo.2019.04.004

62. Kabat-Zinn J. *Wherever You Go, There You Are: Mindfulness Meditation in Everyday Life*. New York: Hyperion; 1994.

63. Segal Z V, Williams JMG, Teasdale JD. *Mindfulness-Based Cognitive Therapy for Depression*. 2nd ed. New York: The Guilford Press; 2013.

64. Simpson R, Simpson S, Ramparsad N, Lawrence M, Booth J, Mercer SW. Mindfulness-based interventions for mental well-being among people with multiple sclerosis: A systematic review and meta-analysis of randomised controlled trials. *J Neurol Neurosurg Psychiatry*. 2019;90(9):1051–1058. https://doi.org/10.1136/jnnp-2018-320165

65. Minden SL, Feinstein A, Kalb RC, et al. Evidence-based guideline: Assessment and management of psychiatric disorders in individuals with MS Report of the Guideline Development Subcommittee of the American Academy of Neurology. *Neurology*. 2014;82(2):174–181. https://doi.org/10.1212/WNL.0000000000000013

66. Fiest KM, Walker JR, Bernstein CN, et al. Systematic review and meta-analysis of interventions for depression and anxiety in persons with multiple sclerosis. *Mult Scler Relat Disord*. 2016;5:12–26. https://doi.org/10.1016/j.msard.2015.10.004

67. Mohr DC, Hart SL, Julian L, Cox D, Pelletier D. Association between stressful life events and exacerbation in multiple sclerosis: A meta-analysis. *Br Med J*. 2004;328(7442):731–733. https://doi.org/10.1136/bmj.38041.724421.55

68. Pagnini F, Bosma CM, Phillips D, Langer E. Symptom changes in multiple sclerosis following psychological interventions: A systematic review. *BMC Neurol*. 2014;14(1):222. https://doi.org/10.1186/s12883-014-0222-z

69. Pagnini F, Phillips D, Bosma CM, Reece A, Langer E. Mindfulness as a protective factor for the burden of caregivers of amyotrophic lateral sclerosis patients. *J Clin Psychol.* 2016;72(1):101–111. https://doi.org/10.1002/jclp.22235

70. Feinstein A, Feinstein K. Depression associated with multiple sclerosis: Looking beyond diagnosis to symptom expression. *J Affect Disord.* 2001;66(2–3):193–198. https://doi.org/10.1016/S0165-0327(00)00298-6

71. Judd LL, Paulus MP, Wells KB, Rapaport MH. Socioeconomic burden of subsyndromal depressive symptoms and major depression in a sample of the general population. *Am J Psychiatry.* 1996;153(11):1411–1417. https://doi.org/10.1176/ajp.153.11.1411

72. Judd LL, Akiskal HS, Maser JD, et al. Major depressive disorder: A prospective study of residual subthreshold depressive symptoms as predictor of rapid relapse. *J Affect Disord.* 1998;50(2–3):97–108. https://doi.org/10.1016/S0165-0327(98)00138-4

73. Silver JM, Yudofsky SC. Aggressive disorders. In: *Neuropsychiatry of Traumatic Brain Injury.* Arlington, VA, US: American Psychiatric Association; 1994:313–353.

74. Eriksson E. Serotonin reuptake inhibitors for the treatment of premenstrual dysphoria. *Int Clin Psychopharmacol.* 1999;14 Suppl 2:S27–33.

75. Prochazka A V., Weaver MJ, Keller RT, Fryer GE, Licari PA, Lofaso D. A randomized trial of nortriptyline for smoking cessation. *Arch Intern Med.* 1998;158(18):2035–2039. https://doi.org/10.1001/archinte.158.18.2035

8. More on Depression and the Causal Complexities of Enduring Sadness

1. Montalban X, Hauser SL, Kappos L, et al. Ocrelizumab versus placebo in primary progressive multiple sclerosis. *N Engl J Med.* 2017;376(3):209–220. https://doi.org/10.1056/NEJMoa1606468

2. Kappos L, Bar-Or A, Cree BAC, et al. Siponimod versus placebo in secondary progressive multiple sclerosis (EXPAND): A double-blind, randomised, phase 3 study. *Lancet.* 2018;391(10127):1263–1273. https://doi.org/10.1016/S0140-6736(18)30475-6

3. Naegelin Y, Naegelin P, Von Felten S, et al. Association of rituximab treatment with disability progression among patients with secondary progressive multiple sclerosis. *JAMA Neurol.* 2019;76(3):274–281. https://doi.org/10.1001/jamaneurol.2018.4239

4. Arnett PA, Higginson CI, Voss WD, Randolph JJ, Grandey AA. Relationship between coping, cognitive dysfunction and depression in multiple sclerosis. *Clin Neuropsychol.* 2002;16(3):341–355. https://doi.org/10.1076/clin.16.3.341.13852

5. Mohr DC, Epstein L, Luks TL, et al. Brain lesion volume and neuropsychological function predict efficacy of treatment for depression in multiple sclerosis. *J Consult Clin Psychol.* 2003;71(6):1017–1024. https://doi.org/10.1037/0022-006X.71.6.1017

6. Mohr DC, Boudewyn AC, Goodkin DE, Bostrom A, Epstein L. Comparative outcomes for individual cognitive-behavior therapy, supportive-expressive group psychotherapy, and sertraline for the treatment of depression in multiple sclerosis. *J Consult Clin Psychol.* 2001;69(6):942–949. https://doi.org/10.1037/0022-006X.69.6.942

7. Chwastiak L, Ehde DM, Gibbons LE, Sullivan M, Bowen JD, Kraft GH. Depressive symptoms and severity of illness in multiple sclerosis: Epidemiologic

study of a large community sample. *Am J Psychiatry*. 2002;159(11):1862–1868. https://doi.org/10.1176/appi.ajp.159.11.1862

8. Patten SB, Lavorato DH, Metz LM. Clinical correlates of CES-D depressive symptom ratings in an MS population. *Gen Hosp Psychiatry*. 2005;27(6):439–445. https://doi.org/10.1016/j.genhosppsych.2005.06.010

9. Minden SL, Orav J, Reich P. Depression in multiple sclerosis. *Gen Hosp Psychiatry*. 1987;9(6):426–434. https://doi.org/10.1016/0163-8343(87)90052-1

10. Ron MA, Logsdail SJ. Psychiatric morbidity in multiple sclerosis: A clinical and MRI study. *Psychol Med*. 1989;19(4):887–895. https://doi.org/10.1017/S0033291700005602

11. Joffe RT, Lippert GP, Gray TA, Sawa G, Horvath Z. Personal and family history of affective illness in patients with multiple sclerosis. *J Affect Disord*. 1987;12(1):63–65. https://doi.org/10.1016/0165-0327(87)90062-0

12. Schiffer RB, Weitkamp LR, Wineman NM, Guttormsen S. Multiple sclerosis and affective disorder: Family history, sex, and HLA-DR antigens. *Arch Neurol*. 1988;45(12):1345–1348. https://doi.org/10.1001/archneur.1988.00520360063013

13. Patten SB, Metz LM, Reimer MA. Biopsychosocial correlates of lifetime major depression in a multiple sclerosis population. *Mult Scler*. 2000;6(2):115–120. https://doi.org/10.1177/135245850000600210

14. IFNB Multiple Sclerosis Study Group. Interferon beta-1b is effective in relapsing-remitting multiple sclerosis. I. Clinical results of a multicenter, randomized, double-blind, placebo- controlled trial. *Neurology*. 1993;43(4 I):655–661. https://doi.org/10.1212/wnl.43.4.655

15. IFNB Multiple Sclerosis Study Group. Interferon beta-lb in the treatment of multiple sclerosis: Final outcome of the randomized controlled trial. *Neurology*. 1995;45(7):1277–1285. https://doi.org/10.1212/WNL.45.7.1277

16. Neilley LK, Goodin DS, Goodkin DE, Hauser SL. Side effect profile of interferon beta-1b in MS: Results of an open label trial. *Neurology*. 1996;46(2):552–554. https://doi.org/10.1212/wnl.46.2.552

17. Mohr DC, Goodkin DE, Likosky W, Gatto N, Baumann KA, Rudick RA. Treatment of depression improves adherence to interferon beta-1b therapy for multiple sclerosis. *Arch Neurol*. 1997;54(5):531–533. https://doi.org/10.1001/archneur.1997.00550170015009

18. Ouallet JC, Radat F, Creange A, et al. Evaluation of emotional disorders before and during treatment with interferon beta in patients with multiple sclerosis. *J Neurol Sci*. 2020;413:116739. https://doi.org/10.1016/j.jns.2020.116739

19. Alba Palé L, León Caballero J, Samsó Buxareu B, Salgado Serrano P, Pérez Solà V. Systematic review of depression in patients with multiple sclerosis and its relationship to interferonβ treatment. *Mult Scler Relat Disord*. 2017;17:138–143. https://doi.org/10.1016/j.msard.2017.07.008

20. Mohr DC, Goodkin DE. Treatment of depression in multiple sclerosis: Review and meta-analysis. *Clin Psychol Sci Pract*. 1999;6(1):1–9. https://doi.org/10.1093/clipsy.6.1.1

21. Feinstein A, O'Connor P, Feinstein K. Multiple sclerosis, interferon beta-1b and depression: A prospective investigation. *J Neurol*. 2002;249(7):815–820. https://doi.org/10.1007/s00415-002-0725-0

22. Gasim M, Bernstein CN, Graff LA, et al. Adverse psychiatric effects of disease-modifying therapies in multiple Sclerosis: A systematic review. *Mult Scler Relat Disord.* 2018;26:124–156. https://doi.org/10.1016/j.msard.2018.09.008

23. Simbrich A, Thibaut J, Khil L, Berger K, Riedel O, Schmedt N. Drug-use patterns and severe adverse events with disease-modifying drugs in patients with multiple sclerosis: A cohort study based on German claims data. *Neuropsychiatr Dis Treat.* 2019;15:1439–1457. https://doi.org/10.2147/NDT.S200930

24. Patten SB, Beck CA, Williams JVA, Barbui C, Metz LM. Major depression in multiple sclerosis: A population-based perspective. *Neurology.* 2003;61(11):1524–1527. https://doi.org/10.1212/01.WNL.0000095964.34294.B4

25. Schiffer RB, Caine ED, Bamford KA, Levy S. Depressive episodes in patients with multiple sclerosis. *Am J Psychiatry.* 1983;140(11):1498–1500. https://doi.org /10.1176/ajp.140.11.1498

26. Bechter K, Reiber H, Herzog S, Fuchs D, Tumani H, Maxeiner HG. Cerebro-spinal fluid analysis in affective and schizophrenic spectrum disorders: Identification of subgroups with immune responses and blood-CSF barrier dysfunction. *J Psychiatr Res.* 2010;44(5):321–330. https://doi.org/10.1016/j.jpsychires.2009.08.008

27. Zunszain PA, Hepgul N, Pariante CM. Inflammation and depression. *Curr Top Behav Neurosci.* 2013;14:135–151. https://doi.org/10.1007/7854_2012_211

28. Rossi S, Studer V, Motta C, et al. Neuroinflammation drives anxiety and depression in relapsing-remitting multiple sclerosis. *Neurology.* 2017;89(13):1338–1347. https://doi.org/10.1212/WNL.0000000000004411

29. Marrie RA, Walld R, Bolton JM et al. Rising incidence of psychiatric disorders before diagnosis of immune-mediated inflammatory disease. *Epidemiol. Psychiatr. Sci.* 2019;28(3):333–342. https://doi.org/10.1017/S2045796017000579

30. Arnett PA, ed. *Secondary Influences on Neuropsychological Test Performance: Research Findings and Practical Applications.* New York: Oxford University Press; 2013.

31. Pujol J, Bello J, Deus J, Martí-Vilalta JL, Capdevila A. Lesions in the left arcuate fasciculus region and depressive symptoms in multiple sclerosis. *Neurology.* 1997;49(4):1105–1110. https://doi.org/10.1212/WNL.49.4.1105

32. Eichert N, Verhagen L, Folloni D, et al. What is special about the human arcuate fasciculus? Lateralization, projections, and expansion. *Cortex.* 2019;118: 107–115. https://doi.org/10.1016/j.cortex.2018.05.005

33. Pujol J, Bello J, Deus J, Cardoner N, Martí-Vilalta JL, Capdevila A. Beck Depression Inventory factors related to demyelinating lesions of the left arcuate fasciculus region. *Psychiatry Res - Neuroimaging.* 2000;99(3):151–159. https://doi .org/10.1016/S0925-4927(00)00061-5

34. Bakshi R, Czarnecki D, Shaikh ZA, et al. Brain MRI lesions and atrophy are related to depression in multiple sclerosis. *Neuroreport.* 2000;11(6):1153–1158. https://doi.org/10.1097/00001756-200004270-00003

35. Feinstein A, Roy P, Lobaugh N, Feinstein K, O'Connor P, Black S. Structural brain abnormalities in multiple sclerosis patients with major depression. *Neurology* 2004;62:586–559. https://doi.org/10.1212/01.wnl.0000110316.12086.0c

36. Gold S, Kern K, O'Connor MF, Montag M, Kim A, Yoo Y, Giesser B, Sicotte N. Smaller cornu ammonis 2–3/dentate gyrus volumes and elevated cortisol in multiple sclerosis patients with depression. *Biological Psychiatry* 2010;68(6):553–559. https://doi.org/10.1016/j.biopsych.2010.04.025

37. Soares J, Marques P, Alves V, Sousa N. A hitchhiker's guide to diffusion tensor imaging. *Frontiers in Neuroscience* 2013;7:1–14. https://doi.org/10.3389/fnins.2013.00031

38. Feinstein A, O'Connor P, Akbar N, Moradzadeh L, Scott CJM, Lobaugh NJ. Diffusion tensor imaging abnormalities in depressed multiple sclerosis patients. *Mult Scler.* 2010;16(2):189–196. https://doi.org/10.1177/1352458509355461

39. Passamonti L, Cerasa A, Liguori M, et al. Neurobiological mechanisms underlying emotional processing in relapsing-remitting multiple sclerosis. *Brain.* 2009;132(Pt 12):3380–3391. https://doi.org/10.1093/brain/awp095

40. Riccelli R, Passamonti L, Cerasa A, et al. Individual differences in depression are associated with abnormal function of the limbic system in multiple sclerosis patients. *Mult Scler.* 2016;22(8):1094–1105. https://doi.org/10.1177/1352458515606987

41. Nigro S, Passamonti L, Riccelli R, et al. Structural "connectomic" alterations in the limbic system of multiple sclerosis patients with major depression. *Mult Scler.* 2015;21(8):1003–1012. https://doi.org/10.1177/1352458514558474

42. Mohr DC, Lovera J, Brown T, et al. A randomized trial of stress management for the prevention of new brain lesions in MS. *Neurology.* 2012;79(5):412–419. https://doi.org/10.1212/WNL.0b013e3182616ff9

43. Shields GS, Spahr CM, Slavich GM. Psychosocial interventions and immune system function: A systematic review and meta-analysis of randomized clinical trials. *JAMA Psychiatry.* 2020;77(10):1031–1043. https://doi.org/10.1001/jamapsychiatry.2020.0431

44. Mohr DC, Hart SL, Julian L, et al. Telephone-administered psychotherapy for depression. *Arch Gen Psychiatry.* 2005;62(9):1007–1014. https://doi.org/10.1001/archpsyc.62.9.1007

45. American Psychological Association. *Diagnostic and Statistical Manual of Mental Disorders.* 4th edition. Washington, DC: American Psychiatric Association; 1994.

46. Schmidt S, Jöstingmeyer P. Depression, fatigue and disability are independently associated with quality of life in patients with multiple sclerosis: Results of a cross-sectional study. *Mult Scler Relat Disord.* 2019;35:262–269. https://doi.org/10.1016/j.msard.2019.07.029

47. Ochoa-Morales A, Hernández-Mojica T, Paz-Rodríguez F, et al. Quality of life in patients with multiple sclerosis and its association with depressive symptoms and physical disability. *Mult Scler Relat Disord.* 2019;36. https://doi.org/10.1016/j.msard.2019.101386

48. Binzer S, McKay KA, Brenner P, Hillert J, Manouchehrinia A. Disability worsening among persons with multiple sclerosis and depression: A Swedish cohort study. *Neurology.* 2019;93(24):E2216–E2223. https://doi.org/10.1212/WNL.0000000000008617

49. McKay KA, Tremlett H, Fisk JD, et al. Psychiatric comorbidity is associated with disability progression in multiple sclerosis. *Neurology.* 2018;90(15):e1316–e1323. https://doi.org/10.1212/WNL.0000000000005302

50. Kalb R, Feinstein A, Rohrig A, Sankary L, Willis A. Depression and suicidality in multiple sclerosis: Red flags, management strategies, and ethical considerations. *Curr Neurol Neurosci Rep.* 2019;19(10):1–8. https://doi.org/10.1007/s11910-019-0992-1

51. Feinstein A, Pavisian B. Multiple sclerosis and suicide. *Mult Scler.* 2017;23(7):923–927. https://doi.org/10.1177/1352458517702553

52. Feinstein A. An examination of suicidal intent in patients with multiple sclerosis. *Neurology*. 2002;59(5):674–678. https://doi.org/10.1212/WNL.59.5.674

53. Mohr DC, Hart SL, Fonareva I, Tasch ES. Treatment of depression for patients with multiple sclerosis in neurology clinics. *Mult Scler*. 2006;12(2):204–208. https://doi.org/10.1191/1352458506ms1265oa

9. Laughter and Tears

1. Feinstein A, Feinstein K, Gray T, O'Connor P. Prevalence and neurobehavioral correlates of pathological laughing and crying in multiple sclerosis. *Arch Neurol*. 1997;54(9):1116–1121. https://doi.org/10.1001/archneur.1997.00550210050012

2. Poeck K. Pathophysiology of emotional disorders associated with brain damage. In: Vinken PJ, Bruyn GW, eds. *Handbook of Clinical Neurology*. Amsterdam: North Holland Publishing Co; 1969;3:343–367.

3. Oppenheim H, Siemerling E. Mitteilungen über Pseudobulbärparalyse und akute Bulbärparalyse. *Berl Kli Woch*, 1886;46:791–794.

4. Wilson SAK. Some problems in neurology, III: Pathological laughing and crying. *J Neurol Psychopathol.*, 1924;4:1299–1333. https://doi.org/10.1136/jnnp.s1-4.16.299

5. Mega MS, Cummings JL, Salloway S, Malloy P. The limbic system: An anatomic, phylogenetic, and clinical perspective. *J Neuropsychiatry Clin Neurosci*. 1997;9(3):315–330. https://doi.org/10.1176/jnp.9.3.315

6. Arciniegas DB, Topkoff J. The neuropsychiatry of pathologic affect: An approach to evaluation and treatment. *Semin Clin Neuropsychiatry*. 2000;5(4):290–306. https://doi.org/10.1053/scnp.2000.9554

7. Ghaffar O, Chamelian L, Feinstein A. Neuroanatomy of pseudobulbar affect: A quantitative MRI study in multiple sclerosis. *J Neurol*. 2008;255(3):406–412. https://doi.org/10.1007/s00415-008-0685-1

8. Wechsler D. *WAIS-R Manual: Wechsler Adult Intelligence Scale–Revised*. Psychological Corporation; 1981.

9. Feinstein A, O'Connor P, Gray T, Feinstein K. Pathological laughing and crying in multiple sclerosis: a preliminary report suggesting a role for the prefrontal cortex. *Mult Scler*. 1999 Apr;5(2):69–73. https://doi.org/10.1177/135245859900500201

10. Hanna J, Feinstein A, Morrow SA. The association of pathological laughing and crying and cognitive impairment in multiple sclerosis. *J Neurol Sci*. 2016;361:200–203. https://doi.org/10.1016/j.jns.2016.01.002

11. Moore SR, Gresham LS, Bromberg MB, Kasarkis EJ, Smith RA. A self report measure of affective lability. *J Neurol Neurosurg Psychiatry*. 1997;63(1):89–93. https://doi.org/10.1136/jnnp.63.1.89

12. Zigmond AS, Snaith RP. The Hospital Anxiety and Depression Scale. *Acta Psychiatr Scand*. 1983;67(6):361–370. https://doi.org/10.1111/j.1600-0447.1983.tb09716.x

13. Schiffer RB, Herndon RM, Rudick RA. Treatment of pathologic laughing and weeping with amitriptyline. *N Engl J Med*. 1985;312(23):1480–1482. https://doi.org/10.1056/NEJM198506063122303

14. McGrane I, VandenBerg A, Munjal R. Treatment of pseudobulbar affect with fluoxetine and dextromethorphan in a woman with multiple sclerosis. *Ann Pharmacother*. 2017;51(11):1035–1036. https://doi.org/10.1177/1060028017720746

15. Johnson B, Nichols S. Crying and suicidal, but not depressed. Pseudobulbar affect in multiple sclerosis successfully treated with valproic acid: Case report and literature review. *Palliat Support Care*. 2015;13(6):1797–1801. https://doi.org/10.1017/S1478951514000376

16. Tortelli R, Copetti M, Arcuti S, et al. Pseudobulbar affect (PBA) in an incident ALS cohort: Results from the Apulia registry (SLAP). *J Neurol*. 2016;263(2):316–321. https://doi.org/10.1007/s00415-015-7981-3

17. Gallagher JP. Pathologic laughter and crying in ALS: A search for their origin. *Acta Neurol Scand*. 1989;80(2):114–117. https://doi.org/10.1111/j.1600-0404.1989.tb03851.x

18. Brooks BR, Thisted RA, Appel SH, et al. Treatment of pseudobulbar affect in ALS with dextromethorphan/quinidine: A randomized trial. *Neurology*. 2004;63(8):1364–1370. https://doi.org/10.1212/01.WNL.0000142042.50528.2F

19. Ban TA. The role of serendipity in drug discovery. *Dialogues Clin Neurosci*. 2006;8(3):335–344. www.dialogues-cns.org. Accessed August 4, 2020.

20. Panitch HS, Thisted RA, Smith RA, et al. Randomized, controlled trial of dextromethorphan/quinidine for pseudobulbar affect in multiple sclerosis. *Ann Neurol*. 2006;59(5):780–787. https://doi.org/10.1002/ana.20828

21. Pioro EP, Brooks BR, Cummings J, et al. Dextromethorphan plus ultra low-dose quinidine reduces pseudobulbar affect. *Ann Neurol*. 2010;68(5):693–702. https://doi.org/10.1002/ana.22093

22. Kappos L, Bar-Or A, Cree BAC, et al. Siponimod versus placebo in secondary progressive multiple sclerosis (EXPAND): A double-blind, randomised, phase 3 study. *Lancet*. 2018;391(10127):1263–1273. https://doi.org/10.1016/S0140-6736(18)30475-6

10. A Break with Reality

1. American Psychological Association (APA). *Diagnostic and Statistical Manual of Mental Disorders*. 5th ed. Washington, DC: American Psychiatric Association; 2013.

2. World Health Organization. *International Classification of Diseases: [9th] Ninth Revision, Basic Tabulation List with Alphabetic Index*. Geneva, Switzerland: World Health Organization; 1978. https://apps.who.int/iris/handle/10665/39473.

3. Patten SB, Svenson LW, Metz LM. Psychotic disorders in MS: Population-based evidence of an association. *Neurology*. 2005;65(7):1123–1125. https://doi.org/10.1212/01.wnl.0000178998.95293.29

4. Marrie RA, Fisk JD, Tremlett H, et al. Differences in the burden of psychiatric comorbidity in MS vs the general population. *Neurology*. 2015;85(22):1972–1979. https://doi.org/10.1212/WNL.0000000000002174

5. Marrie RA, Reingold S, Cohen J, et al. The incidence and prevalence of psychiatric disorders in multiple sclerosis: A systematic review. *Mult Scler J*. 2015;21(3):305–317. https://doi.org/10.1177/1352458514564487

6. Camara-Lemarroy CR, Ibarra-Yruegas BE, Rodriguez-Gutierrez R, Berrios-Morales I, Ionete C, Riskind P. The varieties of psychosis in multiple sclerosis: A systematic review of cases. *Mult Scler Relat Disord*. 2017;12:9–14. https://doi.org/10.1016/j.msard.2016.12.012

7. Aggarwal A, Sharma DD, Kumar R, Sharma RC. Acute psychosis as the initial presentation of MS: A case report. *Int MS J*. 2011;17(2):54–57.

8. Enderami A, Fouladi R, Hosseini SH. First-episode psychosis as the initial presentation of multiple sclerosis: A case report. *Int Med Case Rep J.* 2018;11:73–76. https://doi.org/10.2147/IMCRJ.S157287

9. Zhou Y, Sunwoo M, O'Donoghue B. A case of multiple sclerosis presenting as first-episode psychosis in a young person. *Aust N Z J Psychiatry.* 2020;54(9):942. https://doi.org/10.1177/0004867420910249

10. Gilberthorpe TG, O'Connell KE, Carolan A, et al. The spectrum of psychosis in multiple sclerosis: A clinical case series. *Neuropsychiatr Dis Treat.* 2017;13:303–318. https://doi.org/10.2147/NDT.S116772

11. Feinstein A, Du Boulay G, Ron MA. Psychotic illness in multiple sclerosis. A clinical and magnetic resonance imaging study. *Br J Psychiatry.* 1992;161(NOV.):680–685. https://doi.org/10.1192/bjp.161.5.680

12. Crow TJ, Ball J, Bloom SR, et al. Schizophrenia as an anomaly of development of cerebral asymmetry. A postmortem study and a proposal concerning the genetic basis of the disease. *Arch Gen Psychiatry.* 1989;46(12):1145–1150. https://doi.org/10.1001/archpsyc.1989.01810120087013

13. Suddath RL, Christison GW, Torrey EF, Casanova MF, Weinberger DR. Anatomical abnormalities in the brains of monozygotic twins discordant for schizophrenia. *N Engl J Med.* 1990;322(12):789–794. https://doi.org/10.1056/NEJM199003223221201

14. Radua J, Ramella-Cravaro V, Ioannidis JPA, et al. What causes psychosis? An umbrella review of risk and protective factors. *World Psychiatry.* 2018;17(1):49–66. https://doi.org/10.1002/wps.20490

15. Manfredi G, Kotzalidis GD, Sani G, et al. Persistent interferon-β-1b-induced psychosis in a patient with multiple sclerosis. *Psychiatry Clin Neurosci.* 2010;64(5): 584–586. https://doi.org/10.1111/j.1440-1819.2010.02122.x

16. Lamotte G, Cogez J, Viader F. Interferon-β-1a-induced psychosis in a patient with multiple sclerosis. *Psychiatry Clin Neurosci.* 2012;66(5):462. https://doi.org/10.1111/j.1440-1819.2012.02358.x

17. Warrington TP, Bostwick JM. Psychiatric adverse effects of corticosteroids. *Mayo Clin Proc.* 2006;81(10):1361–1367. https://doi.org/10.4065/81.10.1361

18. Kenna HA, Poon AW, De Los Angeles CP, Koran LM. Psychiatric complications of treatment with corticosteroids: Review with case report. *Psychiatry Clin Neurosci.* 2011;65(6):549–560. https://doi.org/10.1111/j.1440-1819.2011.02260.x

19. Dubovsky AN, Arvikar S, Stern TA, Axelrod L. The neuropsychiatric complications of glucocorticoid use: Steroid psychosis revisited. *Psychosomatics.* 2012;53(2):103–115. https://doi.org/10.1016/j.psym.2011.12.007

20. Lotan I, Fireman L, Benninger F, Weizman A, Steiner I. Psychiatric side effects of acute high-dose corticosteroid therapy in neurological conditions. *Int Clin Psychopharmacol.* 2016;31(4):224–231. https://doi.org/10.1097/YIC.0000000000000122

21. Bloch M, Gur E, Shalev A. Chlorpromazine prophylaxis of steroid-induced psychosis. *Gen Hosp Psychiatry.* 1994;16(1):42–44. https://doi.org/10.1016/0163-8343(94)90086-8

22. Minden SL, Orav J, Schildkraut JJ. Hypomanic reactions to ACTH and prednisone treatment for multiple sclerosis. *Neurology.* 1988;38(10):1631–1634. https://doi.org/10.1212/wnl.38.10.1631

23. Falk WE. Lithium prophylaxis of corticotropin-induced psychosis. *JAMA J Am Med Assoc.* 1979;241(10):1011. https://doi.org/10.1001/jama.1979.03290360 027021

24. Kosmidis MH, Giannakou M, Messinis L, Papathanasopoulos P. Psychotic features associated with multiple sclerosis. *Int Rev Psychiatry.* 2010;22(1):55–66. https://doi.org/10.3109/09540261003589612

25. Hussain A, Belderbos S. Risperidone depot in the treatment of psychosis associated with multiple sclerosis—a case report. *J Psychopharmacol.* 2008;22(8): 925–926. https://doi.org/10.1177/0269881107083997

11. *The Paradox of Time and Space: Redux*

1. Kabat-Zinn J. Mindfulness-based interventions in context: Past, present, and future. *Clin Psychol Sci Pract.* 2003. https://doi.org/10.1093/clipsy/bpg016

decision making: emotion-driven, case history, 143–53; executive function in, 80, 91; saccadic network and, 29

declarative memory, 59

Delis-Kaplan Executive Function System (D-KEFS), 28, 88, 89

DeLuca, J., 70

delusional disorder, 187

delusions, 186, 189, 191

Demirel, S., 6

demyelination, 37, 70, 71

denial, 5, 110

dentate gyrus, 73, 162

depression, 1, 2, 9–10, 118–69; antidepressant therapy, 132, 133–35, 141–42, 180–81, 182; as brain disorder, 73, 159–67; and cognitive impairment, perception of, 67–68; continuum, 118–19; coping strategies and, 124–31, 132–33, 138–39, 153–57; diagnosis, 166–67; disease-modifying therapy and, 157–58; distraction and, 51–52; executive function in, 91; genetic predisposition, 157; hippocampal injury–related, 73; job loss–related, 27; major, 118–19; memory rehabilitation effects, 78; negative effect on cognition, 31, 135–36; neuroimaging studies, 159–65, 167; neuroinflammation-related, 158–60; nonpharmacologic treatment, 31–32, 135–37, 154, 166–67, 180, 201; physical disability–related, 31, 157; problem-solving coping strategy and, 129–30; psychosocial factors, 178–79; psychotherapy for, 138, 180, 195; resilience and, 130–31; as response to MS diagnosis, 120–24; as sadness, 118; self-efficacy and, 131; as steroid-associated mania risk factor, 191; subsyndromal, 139–42; tests for, 180; undertreatment, 168–69

depression case histories: antidepressant therapy, 132–36; diagnosis-related depression, 120–24; dysfunctional coping strategies, 124–29, 132–33, 138–39; irritability, 140–41

despair, 143, 148, 149, 151, 167–68, 175, 193

dextromethorphan-quinidine combination (Nuedexta), 181–83

diagnosis, uncertainty about, 121–22, 124

Diagnostic and Statistical Manual of Mental Disorders (DSM-5), 166, 186–87

diagnostic criteria, 5

diffusion tensor imaging (DTI), 93, 162–63, 164

Digit Span Test, 70; Digits Forward and Digits Backward components, 60, 179

disease-modifying therapies, 56–57, 76, 157–58, 159, 183

distraction, effects on information processing speed, 35–58; depression and, 30–31, 51–52; SDMT performance, 30–31, 46–48, 51–52; and work performance, case histories, 35–44, 48–51

donepezil hydrochloride, 76, 101–2

dorsolateral prefrontal cortex, 29, 92, 164

driving ability, 155

duloxetine, 134, 135

dysarthria, 8, 28–29, 174

educational attainment, 45, 114; case history, 48–51

emotional lability, 172–73; distinguished from pseudobulbar affect, 173–74

emotions, 8; conscious, 175–76; inappropriate display, 177–78; neural connectivity for, 163–64, 176–78; unconscious or involuntary, 176–77

empathy, 103

employment loss, 5–6, 7, 10–11, 130, 197; executive function deficits and, 94–95. *See also* workplace performance case histories

encoding, cognitive, 73, 76–77

episodic memory, 11, 25, 59, 73

episodic memory deficits: assessment, 61–62; case histories, 62–67

European Medicines Agency (EMA), 18

executive function, 80, 92; tests of, 18, 27, 28, 85–89, 179

executive function deficits, 10, 80–97, 154; brain lesion–related, 91–93; case histories, 44, 80–88, 92, 93–94; information processing speed deficits and, 89–90, 95; management strategies, 95–96; memory deficits and, 89–90, 95; prospective memory deficits and, 90; in pseudobulbar affect, 179, 180

exercise, 96–97, 156, 202

Expanded Disability Status Scale (EDSS), 56–57, 129–30, 167, 168, 179

extraversion, 107–8, 111, 114, 115, 116, 130

eye movement abnormalities, 29–30

fantasizing, 199–200

fatigue, 9–10, 23; treatment, 78, 137, 138, 155, 201

financial management capacity, 94

fingolimod, 158

fluoxetine, 134, 180

Food and Drug Administration (FDA), 18–19

Free Verbal Recall test, 70

friendship loss, 5–6, 7; case history, 196–99, 200

frontal lobes/regions, 29, 91–92, 93, 161

frontoparietal region, 93; bilateral, 19

frontotemporal region, 190

Fujimori, Alberto, 185

Gable, Myra, 85–86

Geschwind, Norman, 92–93

ginkgo biloba, 76

glatiramer acetate, 56

globus pallidus, 92

gorilla-in-the-room cognitive test, 52

Grant, David, 85

gray matter, 70–71, 92, 93, 114, 115

guilt, 118, 123

hallucinations, 186, 189, 191

Hamilton Rating Scale for Depression, 133, 134

Harlow, Harry, 85–86

hippocampus: atrophy, 73; demyelinating lesions, 73; in depression, 162, 164; in emotions, 177; in memory and learning functions, 70–71, 72–74, 175; neuron loss, 73; in pseudobulbar affect, 178; sectional anatomy, 73; verbal and visuospatial memory connectivity, 73–74

home care, wheelchair use in, 5

hopelessness, 143

Hospital Anxiety and Depression Scale, 180

humor, 177

hypothalamic-pituitary-adrenal axis, 162

immune-mediated diseases, 31

immune system function, 165–66

impulsivity, 143, 147, 150, 151

inattention blindness, 52

incidental visual memory, 32–34, 54

incontinence, 7, 196–97

information processing, working memory in, 59–60

information processing speed: tests of, 14–15, 16–20, 27, 28, 38–40, 54, 60, 70. See also Symbol Digit Modalities Test

information processing speed deficits, 2, 10, 27, 35–58; depression and anxiety–related, 31; distraction effects, 35–45; executive function deficits and, 89–90; interventions, 16, 56, 78, 96; learning deficits and, 27, 32–34; multitasking and, 35–40

information processing speed deficits, case histories of, 11–48, 154; multitasking, 35–40; time-dependent tasking, 40–45, 50

infracallosal cingulate, 177

inhibitory control, 80

insomnia, 52, 138

Institute of Neurology, London, 189–90

intelligence, 114–15, 179; cognitive reserve and, 44, 45, 48; premorbid (pre-MS), test for, 14–15

intention tremor, 8

interferons, 56, 136–37, 158, 190

interleukins, 159

psychiatric disorders, 96, 159, 186–88
psychosis, 184–94; case history, 184–86, 191–94
psychotherapy, 157. *See also* cognitive behavior therapy; mindfulness-based therapy; supportive-expressive therapy
psychotropic agents, 101, 159, 181–82

quality of life, 5–7; depression and, 168; executive function and, 91; memory rehabilitation effects, 78; mindfulness interventions and, 138; as self-efficacy measure, 131
quetiapine, 191

radiologically isolated syndromes, 9
randomized controlled trials (RCTs): antidepressant medications, 133–35; dextromethorphan-quinidine, 182–83; executive function cognitive rehabilitation, 96; memory aids, 79
Rao, S. M., 9, 27, 70
reading, 14–15, 45
reading tests, 15, 44
recall, 73; tests of, 70
RehaCom program, 78–79, 96
relapse, 188
relapse-remitting MS, 9–10, 11–16; executive function rehabilitation, 96; neuroinflammation, 159; progression, 5, 6
Renoir, P.-A., *Luncheon of the Boating Party*, 198–99, 200
resilience, 124, 131–32
risk continuum, 191
risperidone, 191
rituximab, 148–49
rivastigmine, 76
Ron, Maria, 189–90
Roth, Philip, 119

saccades, 29
Safety, Tolerability, and Efficacy Results (STAR) study, 182–83
scent, emotive power, 176–77
Schiffer, R. B., 133
schizoaffective disorder, 187
schizophrenia, 96, 187–88, 190
Schumacher criteria, 5

secondary progressive MS, 5, 6, 9; dysfunctional coping strategies, 143–54; interventions, 57, 78–79, 154–57, 183
sedatives, 182
Selective Reminding Test, 61–62, 70
selective serotonin reuptake inhibitors (SSRIs), 31–32, 133–34, 141–42, 180
self-assessment, of cognitive dysfunction, 67–70; case history, 68–70
self-efficacy, 131
self-generation strategy, 77
self-testing, 77
semantic memory, 59
sequencing, 80, 84, 85, 91
serendipity, 181–82
sertraline, 31–32, 134, 136
sexuality, 134, 149–50, 180–81, 198, 199–200, 201
Siemerling, E., 174
sildenafil (Viagra), 182
simvastatin, 57
siponimod, 57, 148–49, 183
sleep disturbances, 118, 123, 132, 135
Smiles, Samuel, *Self Help*, 45
social etiquette, 177–78
socialization, 5–6, 7, 155; case history, 195–96
social media, 202
space, paradox of, 6–7, 195–202
spaced learning strategy, 77
spasticity, 7, 108, 124–25, 135
speech impairments, 28–29, 30
steroids, 121, 159, 188–89, 190–91
Story Memory Technique, 77
Story Recall test, 70
Strategy-based Training to Enhance Memory (STEM), 77–78
stress, 13–14, 23, 24; management, 130, 137–38, 164–65, 166
stroke, 96, 174
Stroop Test, 52, 88–89, 92, 179
substance abuse, 187
suicide, 158, 168–69
Sumowski, James, 45
supportive-expressive therapy, 134, 136–37, 154
support systems, 133; absence or loss, 74–76

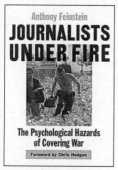
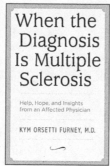
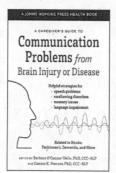
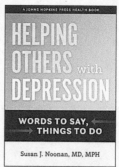
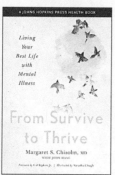
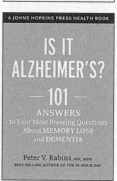
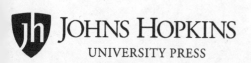
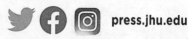